# SOME SPECIAL PROBLEMS IN PERITONEAL DIALYSIS

Edited by **Robert Ekart**

**Some Special Problems in Peritoneal Dialysis**
http://dx.doi.org/10.5772/61982
Edited by Robert Ekart

**Contributors**
Damir Rebić, Vedad Herenda, Desmond Y. H. Yap, Terence Yip, Olga Balafa, Obinna Obinwa, Joseph McLoughlin, Dara Kavanagh, Catherine Wall, David Johnson, Usman Mahmood, Yeoungjee Cho, Guadalupe González, Juan Manuel Gallardo, José Antonio Sanchez-Tomero, Pedro Majano, Elizabeth Flores-Maldonado, Ramón Paniagua, Rafael Selgas, Manuel López Cabrera, Abelardo Isaac Aguilera Peralta, Martin Kimmel, Daniel Kitterer, Joerg Latus, Dominik Alscher, Amarpreet Sandhu, Robert Ekart

**Published by InTech**
Janeza Trdine 9, 51000 Rijeka, Croatia



**Publishing Process Manager** Andrea Koric
**Technical Editor** SPi Global
**Cover** InTech Design team

First published September, 2016
Printed in Croatia

Additional hard copies can be obtained from orders@intechopen.com

Some Special Problems in Peritoneal Dialysis, Edited by Robert Ekart
p. cm.
Print ISBN 978-953-51-2598-3
Online ISBN 978-953-51-2599-0

For EU product safety concerns:
IN TECH d.o.o., Prolaz Marije Krucifikse Kozulić 3, 51000 Rijeka, Croatia,
info@intechopen.com or visit our website at intechopen.com.

# Meet the editor

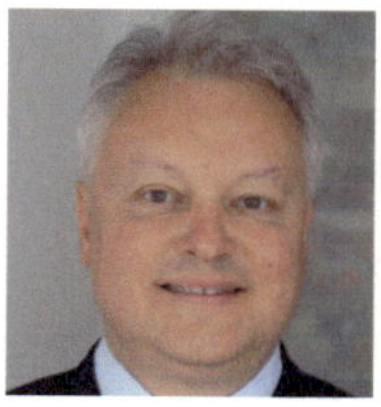

Professor Robert Ekart, MD, born on December 24, 1967, graduated from the Ljubljana Medical School in Slovenia in 1994. He is an associate professor of Internal Medicine at Faculty of Medicine Maribor. Since 2006, he is the Head of the Department of Dialysis in the University Medical Centre Maribor, Slovenia.

He is an active member of ERA-EDTA; a member of ERA-EDTA Scientific Working Groups EURECA-m, DIABESITY, and EUDIAL; board member of the European Journal of Internal Medicine; and reviewer for many international journals (KI, CJASN, AJKD, NDT, AJN, AJH, CKJ, EJIM). His primary research interest is clinical problems in chronic kidney disease and dialysis patients, with emphasis on cardiovascular complications in these patients.

Professor Ekart has published more than 50 papers (PubMed).

# Contents

# Preface

Peritoneal dialysis remains one of the most physiologic, gentle, and home-based forms of dialysis therapy. It is usually provided 24 hours per day and 7 days per week in the form of continuous ambulatory peritoneal dialysis. In this type of peritoneal dialysis, no machine is needed. Another option is automated peritoneal dialysis, in which nightly exchanges are delivered to peritoneal cavity through an automatic peritoneal dialysis cycler. Peritoneal dialysis offers many advantages over hemodialysis, at least during first few years of treatment. There is no need for vascular access; body hydration status and blood chemistry are stable; residual renal function is better preserved in peritoneal dialysis patients than in hemodialysis patients; and the rate of hospitalizations is lower in peritoneal dialysis patients than in hemodialysis patients. One of the most significant advantages of peritoneal dialysis is it is home-based therapy and those who are on peritoneal dialysis have much more free lifestyle with better quality of life than those on hemodialysis.

This book brings the readers some very interesting chapters about peritoneal dialysis.

In the first chapter, we can read an up-to-date, comprehensive review of all types of peritoneal dialysis solutions that are currently available on the market. Dr Johnson et al. discuss conventional peritoneal dialysis solutions and novel solutions with more biocompatible characteristics.

The second chapter by Dr Gónzalez-Mateo introduces us deleterious effects of fibrosis, angiogenesis, lymphangiogenesis, and cell migration on peritoneal membrane preservation. In this section, we can find a special emphasis on the possibility of using drugs capable of preventing or ameliorating peritoneal membrane damage.

Dr Obinwa et al. give us a surgical point of view on peritoneal catheter insertion. They introduce indications and contraindications for peritoneal dialysis, peritoneal dialysis catheter design and materials, the techniques of insertion, complications, and method of removal of dialysis catheters.

In the chapter by Dr Balafa, we can read an up-to-date discussion on the assessment of volume status in peritoneal dialysis patients, including lung comets and bioimpedance techniques.

The chapter by Dr Yap Desmond discusses a very important clinical problem in peritoneal dialysis, exit-site infection of the peritoneal dialysis catheter, which could be a significant cause of peritonitis and catheter loss.

In the chapter by Dr Kimmel, we can read the up-to-date and detailed review about peritoneal dialysis–related infections, including peritonitis, exit-site infections, and tunnel infections.

Dr Rebić discusses in his chapter the suitability of peritoneal dialysis as the method of renal replacement therapy in acute kidney injury patients. The role of peritoneal dialysis in the management of acute kidney injury is, despite new with guidelines from ISPD in 2014, still not well defined, although it remains frequently used in low-resource settings.

The last chapter by Dr Sandhi about peritoneal dialysis and pregnancy is a very exciting chapter with case report and review about details of pregnancy, outcomes, and complications in women on peritoneal dialysis.

I am sure that modern peritoneal dialysis, with its novel solutions, reduced rates of mechanical and infectious complications, and recent survival data, makes peritoneal dialysis the preferred dialysis modality.

I hope that this book will expand the knowledge on peritoneal dialysis and also expand the clinical application of peritoneal dialysis in everyday practice.

I thank Ms. Andrea Koric for her contribution to the secretarial task of collecting and editing the chapters of this book.

**Assoc. Prof. Robert Ekart, MD, PhD**
University Clinical Centre Maribor
Clinic for Internal Medicine
Department of Dialysis
Maribor, Slovenia

Chapter 1

# Introductory Chapter: The Role of Peritoneal Dialysis Today

Robert Ekart

Additional information is available at the end of the chapter

http://dx.doi.org/10.5772/64804

The purpose of this book is to bring the knowledge of many international experts in the field of peritoneal dialysis to readers who have an interest in this type of renal replacement therapy. Unfortunately, in last period the number of patients on peritoneal dialysis in many countries is too small; what has to be taken in mind is the educational process during the period of chronic kidney disease before the start of renal replacement therapy [1]. This process is paramount; as in this period, medical health professionals and patients have enough time for resolving all unclear and unresolved questions.

To make an informed decision on the type of renal replacement therapy, patients should receive timely appropriate education about dialysis options in an educational program covering all modalities. Many patients do not receive such education, and there is a disparity in the information they receive. In the University Clinical Centre Maribor, Clinic for Internal Medicine, Department of Dialysis, Slovenia, we are currently treating 152 patients with the end-stage renal disease. Seventeen of them (11.2%) are on the peritoneal dialysis. One of our patients is being treated with peritoneal dialysis for 13 years; the first method of renal replacement therapy at the beginning has been a few months in-center-hemodialysis.

In February 2015, we began with a systematic, individual predialysis education program of patients with chronic kidney disease who regularly visit nephrology outpatient clinic. Each patient with chronic kidney disease and first seen reduced glomerular filtration rate below 20 ml/min (Stage 4 chronic kidney disease) is redirected to predialysis education. This education is currently implemented only by nurses with specialized knowledge of peritoneal dialysis, who also mastered the hemodialysis treatment. Education is in most patients individual; at the same time, we can educate maximum of up to three patients. My personal belief is that such training must be carried out by nurses who have experience with both peritoneal dialysis and hemodialysis, as well as additional knowledge about kidney transplantation.

Each renal replacement therapy has different advantages and disadvantages, which may make them more or less appropriate for the patient. This depends on his or her clinical and personal situation. Peritoneal dialysis, which requires learning of technical skills by the patient, also requires a degree of responsibility and capability for self-care. Peritoneal dialysis can be performed using several different techniques. The patient could choose between manual exchanges—continuous ambulatory peritoneal dialysis and automated peritoneal dialysis, which use an automated device to do multiple exchanges overnight. The main advantage of peritoneal dialysis is home treatment, and comparing to hemodialysis, peritoneal dialysis gives a much more flexible schedule for different life activities. It is suitable also for older patients with many comorbidities who live at home or in nursing homes. In these patients, it is very important to assist in peritoneal dialysis, which is an evolving dialysis modality. In French and Danish nations, assisted peritoneal dialysis is entirely publicly funded, and the cost of assisted peritoneal dialysis is comparable to the cost of in-center hemodialysis. Assisted continuous ambulatory peritoneal dialysis is the preferred modality in France, whereas assisted automated peritoneal dialysis is the preferred modality in Denmark [2]. Assistants are professional nurses or healthcare technicians briefly educated by expert peritoneal dialysis nurses from the dialysis unit.

There is currently no consensus as to which dialysis modality is the best for elderly patients with end-stage renal disease [3]. In-center hemodialysis is predominant in most countries, although it is widely recognized that peritoneal dialysis has several advantages over hemodialysis, including the lack of need for vascular access, slow continuous ultrafiltration, less interference with patients' lifestyle, and lower costs [3]. In many countries, older end-stage renal disease patients are more rarely initiated on peritoneal dialysis than younger patients. However, greater emphasis should be placed on the promotion of home dialysis therapies such as peritoneal dialysis. Patients should receive balanced and unbiased information about peritoneal dialysis and hemodialysis, including their relative benefits [3]. Dialysis modality choice should be an individual decision, and this choice should be based on the preference of a well-informed and well-prepared patient [3]. Planning of dialysis should be made in advance, whenever possible. A multidisciplinary team should review every patient, aiming to identify potential barriers to peritoneal dialysis and home hemodialysis [3].

This book has been written by widely acknowledged experts, with each chapter providing unique information on some particular problems in the area of peritoneal dialysis. Chapters detail peritoneal dialysis in the acute renal failure, peritoneal dialysis in pregnancy, pharmacological preservation of peritoneal membrane, volume status assessment in peritoneal dialysis patient, microbiologic problems in peritoneal dialysis, surgeon point of view on peritoneal dialysis catheter insertion, and an up-to-date, comprehensive review of all types of peritoneal dialysis solutions that are currently available.

I hope that this book can serve as a resource for expanding the peritoneal dialysis modality in clinical practice.

http://dx.doi.org/10.5772/64804

## Author details

Robert Ekart

Address all correspondence to: robert.ekart2@guest.arnes.si

Department of Dialysis, Clinic for Internal Medicine, University Clinical Centre Maribor, Maribor, Slovenia

## References

[1] Isnard Bagnis C, Crepaldi C, Dean J, Goovaerts T, Melander S, Nilsson EL, et al. Quality standards for predialysis education: results from a consensus conference. Nephrol Dial Transplant. 2015 Jul; 30(7): 1058–1066.

[2] Béchade C, Lobbedez T, Ivarsen P, Povlsen JV. Assisted peritoneal dialysis for older people with end-stage renal disease: the French and Danish experience. Perit Dial Int. 2015 Nov; 35(6): 663–666.

[3] Segall L, Nistor I, Van Biesen W, Brown EA, Heaf JG, Lindley E, et al. Dialysis modality choice in elderly patients with end-stage renal disease: a narrative review of the available evidence. Nephrol Dial Transplant. 2015 Dec 15; pii: gfv411. [Epub ahead of print].

Chapter 2

# Peritoneal Dialysis Solutions

Usman Mahmood, Yeoungjee Cho and
David W. Johnson

Additional information is available at the end of the chapter

http://dx.doi.org/10.5772/63504

**Abstract**

Conventional peritoneal dialysis (PD) solutions are characterized by several undesirable characteristics, including acidic pH (5.2–5.5), high glucose concentrations (13.6–42.5 g/L), hyperosmolarity (360–511 mOsm/kg) and relatively high concentrations of glucose degradation products (GDPs). These characteristics have been shown to result in adverse clinical outcomes, including acute peritoneal membrane toxicity (manifested as inflow pain), chronic peritoneal toxicity (including membrane failure, ultrafiltration failure, peritonitis and encapsulating peritoneal sclerosis) and adverse systemic sequelae (including hyperglycaemia, dyslipidaemia, metabolic syndrome, cardiovascular disease and residual renal function decline). Consequently, there has been a great interest in manufacturing newer solutions with more 'biocompatible' features to mitigate these adverse effects. This has led to the development of neutral-pH, low or ultralow GDP solutions, glucose-sparing PD solutions (icodextrin and amino acid solutions), solutions using alternative osmotic agents (such as hyperbranched polyglycerol) and low-sodium PD solutions. The aim of this chapter is to provide an up-to-date comprehensive review of all types of PD solutions that are currently available, including their impact on patient-level outcomes.

**Keywords:** amino acids, biocompatible materials, controlled clinical trial, dialysis solutions, end-stage kidney disease, glucose, glucose degradation product, glycerol, icodextrin, kidney failure, peritoneal dialysis, polymers, sodium, treatment outcome

## 1. Introduction

Peritoneal dialysis (PD) is a form of renal replacement therapy used to treat patients with end-stage renal disease (ESRD). PD solution is introduced through a peritoneal catheter in the abdomen and replaced either by manual exchanges throughout the day (continuous ambulatory peritoneal dialysis—CAPD) or by a cycler overnight with or without daytime exchanges (automated peritoneal dialysis—APD). PD solutions can be broadly divided into conventional PD solutions and novel solutions with more biocompatible characteristics (e.g. neutral-pH, low glucose degradation products—GDPs solutions). The aim of this chapter is to provide an up-to-date comprehensive review of all types of PD solutions that are currently available, including their impact on patient-level outcomes.

## 2. Conventional PD solutions

During the very early days of PD, the composition of PD solutions varied widely from normal saline to 5% dextrose [1]. Maxwell and colleagues first developed PD solutions akin to currently used conventional PD solutions [2]. Glucose is still being used as the only osmotic agent in PD solutions available for clinical use. Conventional PD solutions contain an osmotic agent (i.e. glucose), lactate as a buffer and electrolytes (i.e. $Na^+$, $Cl^-$, $Ca^{2+}$ and $Mg^{2+}$) (**Table 1**). GDPs, which have been shown to have adverse effects on both the peritoneal membrane and systemically, are produced during the heat sterilization process and/or prolonged storage. This will be discussed later in this chapter.

| PD solution | Manufacturer | pH | Osmotic Agent | Na (mmol/L) | Ca (mmol/L) | Mg (mmol/L) | Lactate (mmol/L) |
|---|---|---|---|---|---|---|---|
| Dianeal | Baxter | 5.5 | Glucose 0.55%, 1.5%, 2.5%, 4.25% | 132 | 1.0/1.25/1.75 | 0.75/0.25 | 35/40 |
| Stay safe | Fresenius | 5.5 | Glucose 1.5%, 2.5%, 4.25% | 134 | 1.25/1.75 | 0.25/0.75 | 35/35 |

PD, peritoneal dialysis.

**Table 1.** Commercially available conventional peritoneal dialysis solution formulations

### 2.1. Osmotic agent—glucose

Conventional PD solutions contain high levels of glucose (dextrose; 75.5–214 mmol/L) as a principal osmotic agent to achieve fluid removal (i.e. ultrafiltration across the peritoneal membrane). Preparations containing different dextrose concentrations (e.g. 0.5 or 0.55%, 1.36 or 1.5%, 2.27 or 2.5% and 3.86 or 4.25% for anhydrous or hydrous dextrose, respectively) are routinely available with varying osmolalities (345–484 mOsm/L). Whilst glucose is a reasonable osmotic agent because it is cheap, easily metabolized, readily available, easily sterilized and associated with an excellent long-term safety profile, the quantity of glucose required for effective ultrafiltration can be problematic. Average systemic glucose absorption from repeated exposure to PD solutions ranges between 100 and 300 g/day [3] (equivalent to 25–75 teaspoons of sugar per day or 36–110 kg/year), depending on dialysate glucose concentration, exchange volume, dwell time and peritoneal transport status. This appreciable peritoneal glucose absorption has in turn been linked with adverse local peritoneal membrane effects and systemic metabolic effects [4]. Glucose in PD solutions triggers protein glycosylation and activates the polyol and protein kinase C pathways [5, 6]. This, along with GDP toxicity and hyperosmolality, potentially results in mesothelial cell death, peritoneal inflammation, neoangiogenesis, epithelial-to-mesenchymal transition (EMT), progressive fibrosis and ultimately peritoneal membrane failure in chronic PD patients [7–11]. Systemic glucose absorption has also been associated with worsening hyperglycaemia in diabetic patients, new-onset hyperglycaemia in incident non-diabetic PD patients, visceral obesity and dyslipidaemia, characterized by elevated levels of total cholesterol, triglyceride, very low-density lipoprotein (VLDL) and low-density lipoprotein (LDL) [12–14]. Consequently, the use of high peritoneal glucose concentrations has been associated with heightened risks of cardiovascular and all-cause mortality [15].

### 2.2. Buffer—lactate

Most of the commercially available conventional PD solutions contain lactate (30–40 mmol/L) as a buffer and are acidic (pH 5.2–5.5). Lactate diffuses into the bloodstream and is rapidly metabolized into bicarbonate. As conventional PD solutions use a single-chamber delivery system, it is not possible to store bicarbonate-buffered solutions, as calcium and bicarbonate will precipitate to form calcium carbonate. Lactate has been shown to inhibit key cellular functions involved in peritoneal defence mechanisms, including phagocytosis, bacterial killing and secretion of cytokines [16].

### 2.3. Electrolyte composition

The concentrations of $Na^+$, $Cl^-$, $Ca^{2+}$ and $Mg^{2+}$ are kept close to those of serum concentrations. Removal of these ions is therefore almost completely dependent on convection due to the low diffusion gradient. For a decilitre of fluid removed in a 4-h dwell, approximately 10 mmol of $Na^+$ and 0.1 mmol of $Ca^{2+}$ are removed, given that serum $Na^+$ and $Ca^{2+}$ are within the reference ranges [17]. Electrolyte concentrations of these solutions vary little by different manufacturers. They are devoid of potassium, and sodium levels mostly range from 132 to 134 mmol/L. Calcium concentrations range from 1.00 to 1.75 mmol/L, depending on the manufacturer (**Table 1**). Patients using calcium-based phosphate binders are recommended to use PD solutions with 1.25 mmol/L [18] calcium concentration to reduce the incidence of hypercalcaemia and adynamic bone disease, which have been previously associated with higher calcium concentrations in PD fluids [19]. The $Mg^{2+}$ concentration is 0.25–0.75 mmol/L. For 1.5%

dextrose solution, 0.25 mmol/L is associated with zero $Mg^{2+}$ transport but for higher glucose concentrations there will be net $Mg^{2+}$ losses, which should be kept in mind.

### 2.4. Glucose degradation products

Several types of GDPs are generated during the heat sterilization process, which are recognized to be toxic at both intra-peritoneal and systemic levels [20, 21]. These include 3-deoxyglucose, 3,4-dideoxyglucosone-3-ene (3,4-DGE), 5-hydroxymethyl furaldehyde, formaldehyde and acetaldehyde. Of the identified GDPs, 3,4-DGE is considered to be the most harmful [22], including its ability to result in dose- and time-dependent renal tubular epithelial cell apoptosis, which raises concern for promoting nephrotoxicity from systemic absorption through PD [23]. Furthermore, various studies have demonstrated adverse effects of these GDPs on peritoneal mesothelial cells, fibroblasts, neutrophils and macrophages, including cytotoxicity, inhibition of proliferation, induction of apoptosis, down-regulation and disturbance of the homeostatic balance of cytokines, and inhibition of migration, bacterial killing, phagocytosis and respiratory burst in phagocytic cells [24–26]. They also promote peritoneal membrane damage and fibrosis, progressive vasculopathy, altered peritoneal transport characteristics, impaired host defence against infections and potentially adverse systemic effects such as increased circulating advanced glycation end products (AGEs) [23, 27, 28].

In summary, conventional PD solutions are characterized by several undesirable characteristics that have been shown to result in adverse clinical outcomes, including peritoneal membrane injury. Consequently, there has been a great interest in manufacturing newer solutions with more 'biocompatible' features in order to mitigate these adverse effects. Subsequent sections of this chapter aim to discuss the current evidence regarding the use of different types of these 'novel' PD solutions and their impact on outcomes.

## 3. Neutral-pH, low GDP PD solutions

Multi-chamber technology has led to the development of neutral-pH, low GDP solutions. Glucose is separated from other electrolytes in one or more chambers and sterilized at a very low pH (2.8–4.2) to minimize the production of GDPs. The remaining solution is kept at an alkaline pH (8.0–8.6) in the other compartment. When PD solution needs to be used, the contents of the two compartments are allowed to mix by breaking a lambda seal or a frangible pin, resulting in the infusion of neutral pH (6.8–7.3), and either a low GDP content (e.g. Physioneal, Baxter Healthcare) or an ultralow GDP content (i.e. less than 80 μmol/L (e.g. Balance or Bicavera, Fresenius Medical Care; Gambrosol Trio, Gambro)) PD solution into the peritoneal cavity. Experimental evidence has reported an improvement in cellular function (e.g. host immune system and peritoneal mesothelial cells), and better preservation of peritoneal membrane from exposure to these solutions [29]. There have been over 20 published randomized controlled trials (RCTs) evaluating the impact of neutral-pH, low GDP solutions on patient-level outcomes [30], and some of their key findings will be summarized in the following sections.

### 3.1. Residual renal function

Treatments using neutral-pH, low GDP solutions have been shown to result in better preservation of residual renal function (11 trials, 643 patients; standardized mean difference (SMD) = 0.17 mL/min; 95% confidence interval (CI), 0.01–0.32; $p$ = 0.04) [31]. Moreover, the benefit was evident across all follow-up durations, extending from less than 6 months (6 trials, 390 patients; SMD: 0.45 mL/min; 95% CI: 0.11–0.79), 6–12 months (9 trials, 568 patients; SMD: 0.24 mL/min; 95% CI: 0.08–0.41) and beyond 12 months in duration (5 trials, 279 patients; SMD: 0.25 mL/min; 95% CI: 0.01–0.48) [31]. Forest plot from cumulative meta-analysis favouring biocompatible PD solutions is shown in **Figure 1**.

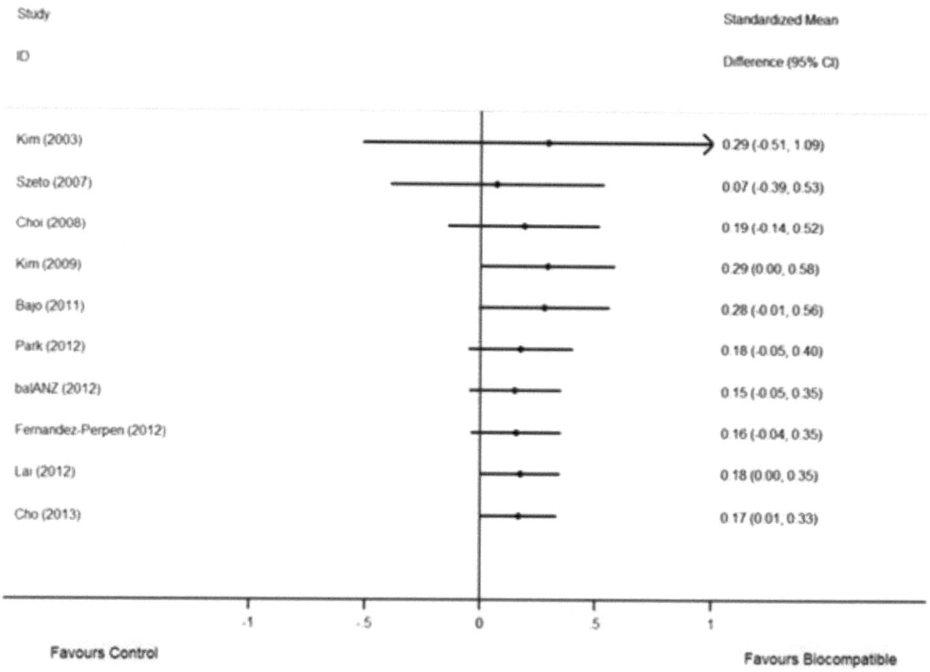


**Figure 1.** Cumulative meta-analysis demonstrating an impact of treatment using neutral-pH, low GDP PD solution on residual renal function (data from randomized controlled trials with follow-up duration greater than or equal to 12 months are included in the analysis) [32–41].

One potential mechanism underlying possible benefit of this solution on residual renal function is reduced systemic absorption of reactive carbonyls (GDPs) from the peritoneal cavity [28]. This could lead to reduced systemic exposure to advanced glycation end products (AGEs), which have been shown to exert direct pro-inflammatory, pro-apoptotic and pro-oxidative nephrotoxicity [23]. In response to the growing level of evidence, the International Society for Peritoneal Dialysis (ISPD) Cardiovascular and Metabolic current guidelines recommend treatments using neutral-pH, low GDP PD solution to better preserve residual renal function in PD patients [42].

### 3.2. Residual urine volume

Similarly, PD treatment using neutral-pH, low GDP solutions has been shown to better preserve residual diuresis (8 trials; 598 patients; mean difference: 127.93 mL/day; 95% CI: 57.54–198.31) [31]. This finding is further supported by previous outcomes from the balANZ trial where the intervention group experienced a significantly lower frequency of anuria (7% vs 20%) and a longer time to onset of anuria ($p = 0.009$) compared to the control group receiving conventional PD solution [38, 43].

### 3.3. Peritoneal ultrafiltration

Although there were concerns that an increase in residual diuresis from treatment using these solutions was a consequence of reduction in ultrafiltration, treatments using neutral-pH, low GDP solutions have not been shown to result in significantly different ultrafiltration when compared to conventional PD solutions (7 trials; 571 patients; mean difference: -110.29 mL/day; 95% CI: -311.67 to 91.09) [31]. Although there has been no RCT conducted to date which measured fluid status objectively (e.g. bioimpedance spectroscopy), clinical findings between patient groups (e.g. body weight, blood pressure) have been shown to be consistently comparable across the various studies [38, 41, 44, 45].

### 3.4. Inflow pain

Inflow pain, which is reported to occur in up to 73% of PD patients, has been attributed to the acidic pH of conventional solutions [29]. The use of neutral-pH solution appears to effectively alleviate this problem [30].

### 3.5. Peritonitis

The balANZ trial has reported a significant benefit in reducing peritonitis risk from treatments using neutral-pH, low GDP PD solutions, with lower peritonitis rates (0.30 vs 0.49 episodes per patient-year) and a significantly longer time to the onset of the first peritonitis episode ($p = 0.01$) [38, 46]. Furthermore, when peritonitis episodes occurred, patients in the intervention group experienced milder symptoms and required shorter hospital duration. Although improved peritoneal host defence mechanisms [46] resulting from exposure to these solutions have been considered as an underlying mechanism, these results have not been similarly replicated by other clinical trials. Nonetheless, none of these trials, including the balANZ trial, was designed to evaluate peritonitis as a primary outcome measure. Interestingly, a meta-analysis was able to demonstrate that some of the heterogeneity that exists amongst the published literature may be driven by the high prevalence of attrition bias (defined as drop-out rate >20%), as the balANZ trial was the only one of the six trials assessed to be at a low risk of attrition bias [47].

### 3.6. Adverse effects

Compared with conventional solutions, biocompatible solutions have not been associated with any harm [30, 47].

### 3.7. Cost

To date, there has only been one economic evaluation of neutral-pH, low GDP PD solutions compared with standard solutions. In a secondary analysis of the balANZ trial, neutral-pH, ultralow GDP PD solution was found to be a cost-effective alternative to standard solutions, primarily as a result of reduction in peritonitis-related hospital costs [48]. Since this time, the costs of biocompatible solutions have fallen significantly, thereby further enhancing their cost-effectiveness.

### 3.8. Other clinical outcomes: peritoneal solute transport and clearance, patient and technique survival

To date, treatments using biocompatible solutions have not been shown to exert a significant impact on outcomes relating to peritoneal solute transport rate, small solute clearance, or patient and technique survival.

### 3.9. Summary

PD using neutral-pH, low GDP PD solution improves clinically important patient-level outcomes, including better preservation of residual renal function, and residual diuresis with probable benefit towards reducing inflow pain. There has been no identified increase in the risk of harm from their use. Moreover, due to recent increase in the uptake of these biocompatible solutions, the cost of therapy has been substantially lowered, and is almost at par with conventional treatments. This has allowed for further increase in uptake in the clinical setting.

## 4. Glucose-sparing strategies

Due to the above-mentioned adverse effects of glucose on the peritoneal membrane as well as its impact at the systemic metabolic level, there has been a great interest in developing strategies for reducing glucose exposure in PD patients. From the PD solution perspective, these options include regular review of the PD prescription to ensure that the glucose strength of PD solution is appropriate and not excessive for an individual patient's needs. A patient's need for peritoneal ultrafiltration (and therefore higher peritoneal glucose concentration) may be further reduced through appropriate dietary salt and water restriction, administration of diuretics and use of strategies to preserve residual renal function (e.g. biocompatible fluids, angiotensin-converting inhibitors or angiotensin receptor blockers, avoidance of hypotension, etc.) [30, 49–53]. An additional option is to use PD solutions that contain non-glucose osmolar agents, such as icodextrin.

## 5. Icodextrin

Icodextrin is a starch-derived, iso-osmolar, high molecular weight (16,200 Daltons) glucose polymer PD solution. The structure of icodextrin is similar to glycogen, consisting of polysaccharide polymers of D-glucopyranose linked by $\alpha$-(1→4) and $\alpha$-(1→6) glucosidic bonds. The pharmacokinetics of icodextrin in blood following intra-peritoneal administration conforms to a simple, single-compartment model that can be approximated by zero-order absorption and first-order elimination [54]. Icodextrin is slowly absorbed via the lymphatics and the resultant osmotic gradient dissipates slowly as compared to glucose, which is absorbed via the small pores of the peritoneal membrane. This provides much greater net ultrafiltration during the long dwell, especially in patients with high transporter status [55, 56]. Treatment using icodextrin has been shown to achieve ultrafiltration equivalent to fluid removal achieved with 4.25% glucose exchange during longer PD dwells (10–16 h) [57]. As such, the ISPD, Australian Icodextrin Consensus Working Group and the European Renal Best Practice (ERBP) Working Group recommend that icodextrin be used for the longer dwell in high transporters with net ultrafiltration of less than 400 mL during a 4-h exchange with a 4.25% dextrose solution [57–59]. The worldwide use of icodextrin has expanded beyond this traditional indication because of accumulating evidence of a favourable benefit:harm profile.

### 5.1. Effects on metabolism: glycaemia and lipid

The glucose-sparing effect of icodextrin has been shown to result in an improvement in metabolic profile based on several observational studies and RCTs [60–62]. The earliest study to demonstrate this was by Johnson et al., who demonstrated significant improvements in the glycaemic control of diabetic PD patients treated with icodextrin, whereby HbA1c levels fell from 8.9 ± 0.7 to 7.9 ± 0.7% [62]. In a subsequent study of 51 diabetic-prevalent patients, the replacement of one of glucose-based PD exchange with icodextrin led to significant reductions in total cholesterol, triglyceride and LDL levels [60]. The reductions were evident as early as 3 months, even though patients were not allowed to initiate or modify existing lipid-lowering treatments for the duration of the study. Similarly, Paniagua and colleagues observed a significant reduction in fasting glucose, insulin requirement, triglyceride and HbA1c levels in those who were randomly assigned to receive icodextrin ($n = 30$) in their multi-centre RCT [61].

### 5.2. Ultrafiltration and fluid status

Icodextrin utilization in a single, daily PD exchange has been shown to increase daily ultrafiltration (4 trials; 103 patients; mean difference: 448.54 mL/day; 95% CI: 289.28–607.80) and reduce episodes of uncontrolled fluid overload without compromising residual renal function (4 trials; 114 patients; standardized mean difference: 0.12, 95% CI: -0.26 to 0.49) [63]. This benefit has been shown to be present for all types of peritoneal membrane transporters, except for those with low transport characteristics [64]. Increases in fluid removal from prescriptions incorporating icodextrin have been shown to objectively improve volume status measured using bioelectrical impedance [65], reduce left ventricular mass index [66], improve ambulatory blood pressure control [67] and significantly reduce episodes of uncontrolled fluid overload (2 trials; 100 patients; relative risk: 0.30; 95% CI: 0.15–0.59) [66].

### 5.3. Patient and technique survival

Despite benefits relating to metabolic profile and fluid status, treatments using icodextrin have not been shown to improve technique (3 trials; 290 patients; relative risk: 0.58; 95% CI: 0.28–1.20) or patient survival [63] (6 trials, 816 patients; relative risk: 0.82; 95% CI: 0.32–2.13). However, the majority of studies included for analysis (more than 60%) had follow-up durations of less than 6 months [63], where one could argue to be too short a follow-up duration to adequately evaluate these outcomes. This, together with the small pooled sample size from studies to date, means that the effects of icodextrin on patient and technique survival remain uncertain.

### 5.4. Adverse effects

Treatments using icodextrin have been shown to increase the serum levels of its metabolites (i.e. maltose and maltotriose), which peak at 2 weeks after treatment commencement and return to normal levels after therapy cessation. Whilst the clinical significance of these metabolite elevations is uncertain, icodextrin is generally recommended to be used in no more than one exchange daily [57]. The accumulation of maltose may lead to overestimation of blood glucose levels due to interference with glucometers using the glucose dehydrogenase pyrroloquinoline quinone (GDH PQQ) method, such that patients may experience hypoglycaemia through inadvertent excessive insulin administration [68]. Guidelines therefore recommend that diabetic PD patients using icodextrin should perform blood sugar measurements using a glucose-specific method (e.g. glucose oxidase or hexokinase reference methods) [57]. Other potential risks from icodextrin use include skin rash, which can lead to therapy cessation (0–4.3% of patients) [69], and sterile peritonitis, which fortunately has not been problematic since the introduction of quality assurance programme monitoring of peptidoglycan levels [55].

### 5.5. Twice daily icodextrin

The use of twice daily icodextrin (8 h/exchange) has been proposed to take advantage of its glucose-sparing characteristics and high ultrafiltration efficiency. Not surprisingly, the studies have reported a reduction in glucose exposure, better ultrafiltration and blood pressure control with an improvement in cardiac parameters on echocardiogram [70–73]. However, all studies to date had small sample sizes and short follow-up durations (<6 months). Furthermore, the product information of icodextrin still recommends its use to be limited as a single exchange in each 24-h period as insufficient safety data are available on the effects of more frequent administration. Therefore, the routine use of twice daily icodextrin cannot be recommended until further data are available on safety and efficacy.

### 5.6. Summary

PD incorporating a single daily exchange of icodextrin results in significantly higher ultrafiltration, which leads to improvement in volume status and cardiac parameters, without adversely affecting residual renal function. Although there has been no convincing evidence to suggest an improvement in technique or patient survival from its use and icodextrin is more costly than conventional PD solutions, the utilization of icodextrin is likely to be a more cost-effective option in patients with ultrafiltration failure than transferring to haemodialysis.

## 6. Amino acid solutions

Peritoneal dialysis causes loss of protein and amino acids in the dialysate, which contributes to the development of protein and energy malnutrition in these patients. Amino acid solutions were developed with an aim to compensate for protein loss. These products are osmotically equivalent to 1.5% glucose PD solutions, although their use is limited to a single daily exchange due to a risk of worsening systemic acidosis and uraemia [74]. Amino acid PD solutions have been shown to improve surrogate markers of nutritional status (e.g. insulin-like growth factor-1, pre-albumin, transferrin) in malnourished PD patients over a 3-month period [75]. However, a subsequent 3-year RCT did not show any significant impact of amino acid PD solution on hospitalization or mortality in 60 malnourished PD patients. Therefore, the role of amino acid solutions remains uncertain in the absence of evidence relating to impact on patient-level clinical outcomes.

## 7. Combination glucose- and GDP-sparing solutions

More recently, there has been an interest in combining icodextrin, amino acid and neutral-pH, low GDP PD solutions as part of glucose-sparing PD therapy. The most recent and the largest RCT conducted was the IMPENDIA-EDEN study [76]. This was an open-label, parallel design trial combining two studies which in total randomized 127 patients to glucose only, and 124 to glucose-sparing treatment group (i.e. one exchange of amino acid PD solution, one exchange of icodextrin and two exchanges of glucose-based PD solutions) for 6 months. The primary outcome measure was a change in HbA1c from baseline. During the study, there was a significant decrease in the mean HbA1c in the glucose-sparing arm with a mean difference of 0.5% between the two groups ($p$ = 0.006) [76]. However, patients in the glucose-sparing group experienced a significantly higher frequency of serious adverse events (105 vs 78) and more deaths (11 vs 5). A large proportion of these events were from fluid overload and hypertensive encephalopathy. This was an unexpected outcome as the glucose-sparing group received icodextrin, which is known to increase ultrafiltration. Later, the study investigators hypothesized that some participating centres attempted to overachieve HbA1c reduction at the expense of peritoneal ultrafiltration by inappropriately reducing the glucose strength of glucose-based PD solutions in the intervention group, which led to this devastating consequence.

In summary, glucose-sparing PD therapy has been shown to improve metabolic profile (i.e. glycaemic control and lipid profile). However, there are residual concerns about its safety, and therefore its use cannot be widely recommended at present **Figure 2**.

http://dx.doi.org/10.5772/63504

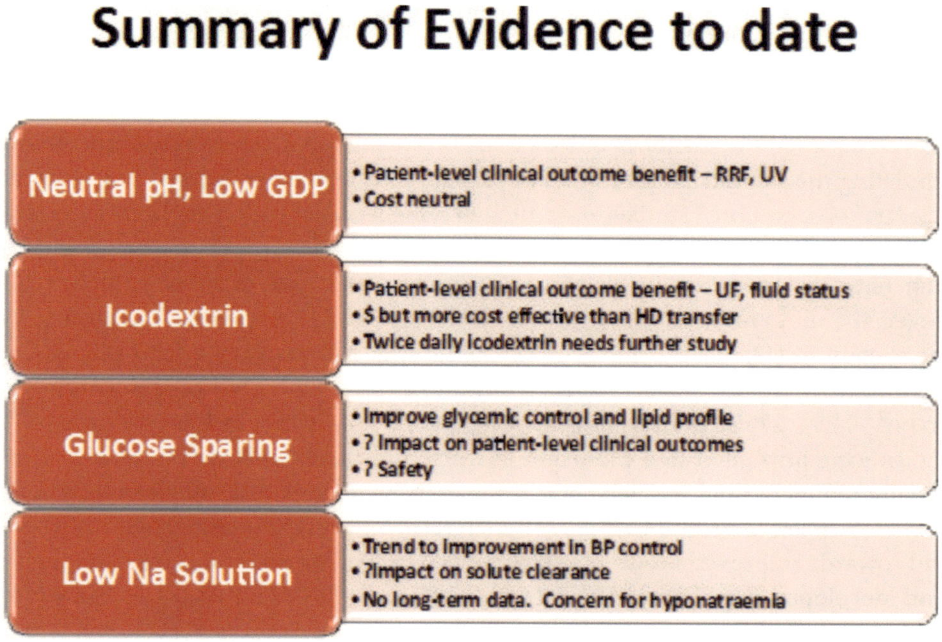


**Figure 2.** Current evidence regarding available PD solutions. RRF (residual renal function), UV (urine volume), UF (ultrafiltration), and HD (haemodialysis).

## 8. PD solutions: future

The ideal PD solution should have a physiologic electrolyte and buffer composition and have an osmotic agent that is non-toxic, non-immunogenic, and not be rapidly absorbed into the plasma compartment (or, if it is, it should ideally be rapidly metabolized). Furthermore, it should produce steady osmotic ultrafiltration over the course of a dwell. So far, glucose has been the universally used osmotic agent in peritoneal dialysis, based on its relative efficiency, low cost, safety and rapid metabolism in plasma. There has been a great interest in developing new osmotic agents that meet the above criteria. One such new agent is hyperbranched polyglycerol (HPG) [77], a branched compact polyether polymer (glycidol monomer). As an osmotic agent, HPG fulfills the criteria of being ideal in size and physical properties and appears to be non-toxic, non-immunogenic and highly biocompatible. It can be manufactured with different molecular weights to add in further flexibility if it is to be implemented in future clinical practice. About 60% is retained in the peritoneum but 25% is excreted in urine. However, its long-term safety, biocompatibility, metabolism and plasma accumulation during long-term use remains unknown and is currently in the preclinical evaluation phase. Other osmotic agents, which have been studied, include L-carnitine and alanyl-glutamine, but none of these solutions are currently available for clinical use.

Another type of PD solution currently undergoing further assessment is low-sodium PD solutions. The rationales for low-sodium PD solution are (i) to increase absolute sodium removal for a given glucose load and (ii) to reduce the 'gap' between sodium and water removal (a consequence of sodium sieving via the aquaporin pathway). As volume homeostasis is an important predictor of outcome in PD patients, an increase in sodium removal by manipulating the sodium concentration of PD solutions to increase net sodium loss is attractive. Several observational studies examining varying levels of sodium concentration (98–120 mmol/L), either as a single exchange or four exchanges daily, have shown an increase in sodium removal, reduction in blood pressure and a decrease in thirst response [78–80]. However, the most recent multi-centre, multinational RCT comparing low-sodium versus standard sodium (125 vs 134 mmol/L) PD solution in hypertensive CAPD patients over 6 month follow-up duration observed an inferior total Kt/V with low-sodium solution (mean difference -0.78), whilst peritoneal Kt/V was comparable between the two groups. These outcomes were attributed to a reduction in thirst and fluid intake in the treatment group, potentially reducing fluid overload and urine excretion (similar to salt-restricted diet intervention), which led to a significant reduction in renal Kt/V in the treatment group. There was a trend towards improved blood pressure control in the low-sodium group although more patients developed hyponatraemia than the control group [81]. In light of the paucity of evidence to date and the presence of some safety signals, low-sodium PD solutions cannot be routinely recommended for clinical practice at this stage.

## 9. Conclusions

None of the currently available PD solutions is perfect. The PD community needs to remain vigilant in its efforts to develop solutions that are more 'biocompatible', ideally using a non-glucose osmolar agent, which is non-toxic, easily metabolized, easily manufactured, cost-effective and metabolically efficient (i.e. predictable ultrafiltration profile with large ultrafiltration volume per unit mass absorption). Experimental models and international collaboration are required to advance this field of research. In the meantime, individualizing therapy to account for particular patient characteristics is necessary to improve clinical outcomes.

## Author details

Usman Mahmood[1], Yeoungjee Cho[1,2] and David W. Johnson[1,2*]

*Address all correspondence to: david.johnson2@health.qld.gov.au

1 Department of Nephrology, Princess Alexandra Hospital, Brisbane, Australia

2 Centre for Kidney Disease Research, Translational Research Institute, University of Queensland, Brisbane, Australia

## References

[1] Oreopoulos DG TE. The history of peritoneal dialysis: early years of Toronto Western Hospital. Dialysis & Transplantation. 2010;39(8):338–43.

[2] Maxwell MH, Rockney RE, Kleeman CR, Twiss MR. Peritoneal dialysis. 1. Technique and applications. Journal of the American Medical Association. 1959;170(8):917–24.

[3] Szeto CC, Chow KM, Kwan BC, Chung KY, Leung CB, Li PK. New-onset hyperglycemia in nondiabetic chinese patients started on peritoneal dialysis. American Journal of Kidney Diseases: The Official Journal of the National Kidney Foundation. 2007;49(4): 524–32.

[4] Holmes CJ. Reducing cardiometabolic risk in peritoneal dialysis patients: role of the dialysis solution. Journal of Diabetes Science and Technology. 2009;3(6): 1472–80.

[5] Ha H, Yu MR, Lee HB. High glucose-induced PKC activation mediates TGF-beta 1 and fibronectin synthesis by peritoneal mesothelial cells. Kidney International. 2001;59(2): 463–70.

[6] Lee HB, Yu MR, Song JS, Ha H. Reactive oxygen species amplify protein kinase C signaling in high glucose-induced fibronectin expression by human peritoneal mesothelial cells. Kidney International. 2004;65(4):1170–9.

[7] Mortier S, De Vriese AS, Van de Voorde J, Schaub TP, Passlick-Deetjen J, Lameire NH. Hemodynamic effects of peritoneal dialysis solutions on the rat peritoneal membrane: role of acidity, buffer choice, glucose concentration, and glucose degradation products. Journal of the American Society of Nephrology: JASN. 2002;13(2):480–9.

[8] Devuyst O, Topley N, Williams JD. Morphological and functional changes in the dialysed peritoneal cavity: impact of more biocompatible solutions. Nephrology, Dialysis, Transplantation: Official Publication of the European Dialysis and Transplant Association – European Renal Association. 2002;17 Suppl 3:12–5.

[9] Davies SJ, Phillips L, Naish PF, Russell GI. Peritoneal glucose exposure and changes in membrane solute transport with time on peritoneal dialysis. Journal of the American Society of Nephrology: JASN. 2001;12(5):1046–51.

[10] Wu HY, Hung KY, Huang JW, Chen YM, Tsai TJ, Wu KD. Initial glucose load predicts technique survival in patients on chronic peritoneal dialysis. American Journal of Nephrology. 2008;28(5):765–71.

[11] Wu HY, Hung KY, Huang TM, Hu FC, Peng YS, Huang JW, et al. Safety issues of long-term glucose load in patients on peritoneal dialysis – a 7-year cohort study. PloS One. 2012;7(1):e30337.

[12] Holmes CJ, Shockley TR. Strategies to reduce glucose exposure in peritoneal dialysis patients. Peritoneal Dialysis International: Journal of the International Society for Peritoneal Dialysis. 2000;20 Suppl 2:S37–41.

[13] Holmes C, Mujais S. Glucose sparing in peritoneal dialysis: implications and metrics. Kidney International Supplement. 2006; 70 (Suppl 103):S104–9.

[14] Cotovio P, Rocha A, Rodrigues A. Peritoneal dialysis in diabetics: there is room for more. International Journal of Nephrology. 2011;2011:914849.

[15] Wen Y, Guo Q, Yang X, Wu X, Feng S, Tan J, et al. High glucose concentrations in peritoneal dialysate are associated with all-cause and cardiovascular disease mortality in continuous ambulatory peritoneal dialysis patients. Peritoneal Dialysis International: Journal of the International Society for Peritoneal Dialysis. 2015;35(1):70–7.

[16] Schambye HT. Effect of different buffers on the biocompatibility of CAPD solutions. Peritoneal Dialysis International: Journal of the International Society for Peritoneal Dialysis. 1996;16 Suppl 1:S130–6.

[17] Rippe B, Venturoli D, Simonsen O, de Arteaga J. Fluid and electrolyte transport across the peritoneal membrane during CAPD according to the three-pore model. Peritoneal Dialysis International: Journal of the International Society for Peritoneal Dialysis. 2004;24(1):10–27.

[18] Johnson DW, Rigby RJ, McIntyre HD, Brown A, Freeman J. A randomized trial comparing 1.25 mmol/l calcium dialysate to 1.75 mmol/l calcium dialysate in CAPD patients. Nephrology, Dialysis, Transplantation: Official Publication of the European Dialysis and Transplant Association – European Renal Association. 1996;11(1):88–93.

[19] Haris A, Sherrard DJ, Hercz G. Reversal of adynamic bone disease by lowering of dialysate calcium. Kidney International. 2006;70(5):931–7.

[20] Nilsson-Thorell CB, Muscalu N, Andren AH, Kjellstrand PT, Wieslander AP. Heat sterilization of fluids for peritoneal dialysis gives rise to aldehydes. Peritoneal Dialysis International: Journal of the International Society for Peritoneal Dialysis. 1993;13(3): 208–13.

[21] Catalan MP, Santamaria B, Reyero A, Ortiz A, Egido J, Ortiz A. 3,4-di-deoxyglucosone-3-ene promotes leukocyte apoptosis. Kidney International. 2005;68(3):1303–11.

[22] Erixon M, Wieslander A, Linden T, Carlsson O, Forsback G, Svensson E, et al. How to avoid glucose degradation products in peritoneal dialysis fluids. Peritoneal Dialysis International: Journal of the International Society for Peritoneal Dialysis. 2006;26(4): 490–7.

[23] Justo P, Sanz AB, Egido J, Ortiz A. 3,4-Dideoxyglucosone-3-ene induces apoptosis in renal tubular epithelial cells. Diabetes. 2005;54(8):2424–9.

[24] Witowski J, Korybalska K, Ksiazek K, Wisniewska-Elnur J, Jorres A, Lage C, et al. Peritoneal dialysis with solutions low in glucose degradation products is associated

with improved biocompatibility profile towards peritoneal mesothelial cells. Nephrology, Dialysis, Transplantation: Official Publication of the European Dialysis and Transplant Association – European Renal Association. 2004;19(4):917–24.

[25] Jonasson P, Albrektsson A, Ljungman S, Wieslander A, Braide M. Peritoneal leukocyte survival and respiratory burst responses in patients treated with a low glucose degradation and high pH peritoneal dialysis fluid. The International Journal of Artificial Organs. 2003;26(2):121–8.

[26] Wieslander AP, Nordin MK, Martinson E, Kjellstrand PT, Boberg UC. Heat sterilized PD-fluids impair growth and inflammatory responses of cultured cell lines and human leukocytes. Clinical Nephrology. 1993;39(6):343–8.

[27] Mortier S, Faict D, Schalkwijk CG, Lameire NH, De Vriese AS. Long-term exposure to new peritoneal dialysis solutions: effects on the peritoneal membrane. Kidney International. 2004;66(3):1257–65.

[28] Zeier M, Schwenger V, Deppisch R, Haug U, Weigel K, Bahner U, et al. Glucose degradation products in PD fluids: do they disappear from the peritoneal cavity and enter the systemic circulation? Kidney International. 2003;63(1):298–305.

[29] Boulanger E, Wautier MP, Wautier JL, Boval B, Panis Y, Wernert N, et al. AGEs bind to mesothelial cells via RAGE and stimulate VCAM-1 expression. Kidney International. 2002;61(1):148–56.

[30] Cho Y, Johnson DW, Craig JC, Strippoli GF, Badve SV, Wiggins KJ. Biocompatible dialysis fluids for peritoneal dialysis. The Cochrane Database of Systematic Reviews. 2014;3:Cd007554.

[31] Yohanna S, Alkatheeri AM, Brimble SK, McCormick B, Iansavitchous A, Blake PG, et al. Effect of neutral-pH, low-glucose degradation product peritoneal dialysis solutions on residual renal function, urine volume, and ultrafiltration: asystematic review and meta-analysis. Clinical Journal of the American Society of Nephrology: CJASN. 2015;10(8):1380–8.

[32] Choi HY, Kim DK, Lee TH, Moon SJ, Han SH, Lee JE, et al. The clinical usefulness of peritoneal dialysis fluids with neutral pH and low glucose degradation product concentration: an open randomized prospective trial. Peritoneal Dialysis International: Journal of the International Society for Peritoneal Dialysis. 2008;28(2):174–82.

[33] Szeto CC, Chow KM, Lam CW, Leung CB, Kwan BC, Chung KY, et al. Clinical biocompatibility of a neutral peritoneal dialysis solution with minimal glucose-degradation products – a 1-year randomized control trial. Nephrology, Dialysis, Transplantation: Official Publication of the European Dialysis and Transplant Association – European Renal Association. 2007;22(2):552–9.

[34] Cho KH, Do JY, Park JW, Yoon KW, Kim YL. The effect of low-GDP solution on ultrafiltration and solute transport in continuous ambulatory peritoneal dialysis

patients. Peritoneal Dialysis International: Journal of the International Society for Peritoneal Dialysis. 2013;33(4):382–90.

[35] Bajo MA, Perez-Lozano ML, Albar-Vizcaino P, del Peso G, Castro MJ, Gonzalez-Mateo G, et al. Low-GDP peritoneal dialysis fluid ('balance') has less impact in vitro and ex vivo on epithelial-to-mesenchymal transition (EMT) of mesothelial cells than a standard fluid. Nephrology, Dialysis, Transplantation: Official Publication of the European Dialysis and Transplant Association – European Renal Association. 2011;26(1):282–91.

[36] Park SH, Do JY, Kim YH, Lee HY, Kim BS, Shin SK, et al. Effects of neutral pH and low-glucose degradation product-containing peritoneal dialysis fluid on systemic markers of inflammation and endothelial dysfunction: a randomized controlled 1-year follow-up study. Nephrology, Dialysis, Transplantation: Official Publication of the European Dialysis and Transplant Association – European Renal Association. 2012;27(3):1191–9.

[37] Lai KN, Lam MF, Leung JC, Chan LY, Lam CW, Chan IH, et al. A study of the clinical and biochemical profile of peritoneal dialysis fluid low in glucose degradation products. Peritoneal Dialysis International: Journal of the International Society for Peritoneal Dialysis. 2012;32(3):280–91.

[38] Johnson DW, Brown FG, Clarke M, Boudville N, Elias TJ, Foo MW, et al. Effects of biocompatible versus standard fluid on peritoneal dialysis outcomes. Journal of the American Society of Nephrology: JASN. 2012;23(6):1097–107.

[39] Fernandez-Perpen A, Perez-Lozano ML, Bajo MA, Albar-Vizcaino P, Sandoval Correa P, del Peso G, et al. Influence of bicarbonate/low-GDP peritoneal dialysis fluid (BicaVera) on in vitro and ex vivo epithelial-to-mesenchymal transition of mesothelial cells. Peritoneal Dialysis International: Journal of the International Society for Peritoneal Dialysis. 2012;32(3):292–304.

[40] Kim YL, Do J, Park SH, Cho K, Park J, Yoon K, et al. Low glucose degradation products dialysis solution modulates the levels of surrogate markers of peritoneal inflammation, integrity, and angiogenesis: preliminary report. Nephrology (Carlton, Vic). 2003;8 Suppl:S28–32.

[41] Kim S, Oh J, Kim S, Chung W, Ahn C, Kim SG, et al. Benefits of biocompatible PD fluid for preservation of residual renal function in incident CAPD patients: a 1-year study. Nephrology, Dialysis, Transplantation: Official Publication of the European Dialysis and Transplant Association – European Renal Association. 2009;24(9):2899–908.

[42] Wang AY, Brimble KS, Brunier G, Holt SG, Jha V, Johnson DW, et al. ISPD Cardiovascular and metabolic guidelines in adult peritoneal dialysis patients part I –assessment and management of various cardiovascular risk factors. Peritoneal Dialysis International: Journal of the International Society for Peritoneal Dialysis. 2015;35(4):379–87.

[43] Johnson DW, Brown FG, Clarke M, Boudville N, Elias TJ, Foo MW, et al. The effect of low glucose degradation product, neutral pH versus standard peritoneal dialysis

solutions on peritoneal membrane function: the balANZ trial. Nephrology, Dialysis, Transplantation: Official Publication of the European Dialysis and Transplant Association – European Renal Association. 2012;27(12):4445–53.

[44] Kim SG, Kim S, Hwang YH, Kim K, Oh JE, Chung W, et al. Could solutions low in glucose degradation products preserve residual renal function in incident peritoneal dialysis patients? A 1-year multicenter prospective randomized controlled trial (Balnet Study). Peritoneal Dialysis International: Journal of the International Society for Peritoneal Dialysis. 2008;28 Suppl 3:S117–22.

[45] Fan SL, Pile T, Punzalan S, Raftery MJ, Yaqoob MM. Randomized controlled study of biocompatible peritoneal dialysis solutions: effect on residual renal function. Kidney International. 2008;73(2):200–6.

[46] Johnson DW, Brown FG, Clarke M, Boudville N, Elias TJ, Foo MW, et al. The effects of biocompatible compared with standard peritoneal dialysis solutions on peritonitis microbiology, treatment, and outcomes: the balANZ trial. Peritoneal Dialysis International: Journal of the International Society for Peritoneal Dialysis. 2012;32(5):497–506.

[47] Cho Y, Johnson DW, Badve SV, Craig JC, Strippoli GF, Wiggins KJ. The impact of neutral-pH peritoneal dialysates with reduced glucose degradation products on clinical outcomes in peritoneal dialysis patients. Kidney International. 2013;84(5):969–79.

[48] Howard K, Hayes A, Cho Y, Cass A, Clarke M, Johnson DW. Economic evaluation of neutral-pH, low-glucose degradation product peritoneal dialysis solutions compared with standard solutions: a secondary analysis of the balANZ Trial. American Journal of Kidney Diseases: The Official Journal of the National Kidney Foundation. 2015;65(5):773–9.

[49] Quan L, Xu Y, Luo SP, Wang L, LeBlanc D, Wang T. Negotiated care improves fluid status in diabetic peritoneal dialysis patients. Peritoneal Dialysis International: Journal of the International Society for Peritoneal Dialysis. 2006;26(1):95–100.

[50] Gan HB, Chen MH, Lindholm B, Wang T. Volume control in diabetic and nondiabetic peritoneal dialysis patients. International Urology and Nephrology. 2005;37(3):575–9.

[51] Li PK, Chow KM, Wong TY, Leung CB, Szeto CC. Effects of an angiotensin-converting enzyme inhibitor on residual renal function in patients receiving peritoneal dialysis. A randomized, controlled study. Annals of Internal Medicine. 2003;139(2):105–12.

[52] Suzuki H, Kanno Y, Sugahara S, Okada H, Nakamoto H. Effects of an angiotensin II receptor blocker, valsartan, on residual renal function in patients on CAPD. American Journal of Kidney Diseases: The Official Journal of the National Kidney Foundation. 2004;43(6):1056–64.

[53] Medcalf JF, Harris KP, Walls J. Role of diuretics in the preservation of residual renal function in patients on continuous ambulatory peritoneal dialysis. Kidney International. 2001;59(3):1128–33.

[54] Moberly JB, Mujais S, Gehr T, Hamburger R, Sprague S, Kucharski A, et al. Pharmacokinetics of icodextrin in peritoneal dialysis patients. Kidney International Supplement. 2002(81):S23–33.

[55] Silver SA, Harel Z, Perl J. Practical considerations when prescribing icodextrin: a narrative review. American Journal of Nephrology. 2014;39(6):515–27.

[56] Wiggins KJ, Rumpsfeld M, Blizzard S, Johnson DW. Predictors of a favourable response to icodextrin in peritoneal dialysis patients with ultrafiltration failure. Nephrology (Carlton, Vic). 2005;10(1):33–6.

[57] Johnson DW, Agar J, Collins J, Disney A, Harris DC, Ibels L, et al. Recommendations for the use of icodextrin in peritoneal dialysis patients. Nephrology (Carlton, Vic). 2003;8(1):1–7.

[58] Mujais S, Nolph K, Gokal R, Blake P, Burkart J, Coles G, et al. Evaluation and management of ultrafiltration problems in peritoneal dialysis. International Society for Peritoneal Dialysis Ad Hoc Committee on Ultrafiltration Management in Peritoneal Dialysis. Peritoneal Dialysis International: Journal of the International Society for Peritoneal Dialysis. 2000;20 Suppl 4:S5–21.

[59] van Biesen W, Heimburger O, Krediet R, Rippe B, La Milia V, Covic A, et al. Evaluation of peritoneal membrane characteristics: clinical advice for prescription management by the ERBP working group. Nephrology, Dialysis, Transplantation: Official Publication of the European Dialysis and Transplant Association – European Renal Association. 2010;25(7):2052–62.

[60] Babazono T, Nakamoto H, Kasai K, Kuriyama S, Sugimoto T, Nakayama M, et al. Effects of icodextrin on glycemic and lipid profiles in diabetic patients undergoing peritoneal dialysis. American Journal of Nephrology. 2007;27(4):409–15.

[61] Paniagua R, Ventura MD, Avila-Diaz M, Cisneros A, Vicente-Martinez M, Furlong MD, et al. Icodextrin improves metabolic and fluid management in high and high-average transport diabetic patients. Peritoneal Dialysis International: Journal of the International Society for Peritoneal Dialysis. 2009;29(4):422–32.

[62] Johnson DW, Arndt M, O'Shea A, Watt R, Hamilton J, Vincent K. Icodextrin as salvage therapy in peritoneal dialysis patients with refractory fluid overload. BMC Nephrology. 2001;2:2.

[63] Cho Y, Johnson DW, Badve S, Craig JC, Strippoli GF, Wiggins KJ. Impact of icodextrin on clinical outcomes in peritoneal dialysis: a systematic review of randomized controlled trials. Nephrology, Dialysis, Transplantation: Official Publication of the European Dialysis and Transplant Association – European Renal Association. 2013;28(7):1899–907.

[64] Qi H, Xu C, Yan H, Ma J. Comparison of icodextrin and glucose solutions for long dwell exchange in peritoneal dialysis: a meta-analysis of randomized controlled trials. Peritoneal Dialysis International: Journal of the International Society for Peritoneal Dialysis. 2011;31(2):179–88.

[65] Davies SJ, Woodrow G, Donovan K, Plum J, Williams P, Johansson AC, et al. Icodextrin improves the fluid status of peritoneal dialysis patients: results of a double-blind randomized controlled trial. Journal of the American Society of Nephrology: JASN. 2003;14(9):2338–44.

[66] Konings CJ, Kooman JP, Schonck M, Gladziwa U, Wirtz J, van den Wall Bake AW, et al. Effect of icodextrin on volume status, blood pressure and echocardiographic parameters: a randomized study. Kidney International. 2003;63(4):1556–63.

[67] Paniagua R, Orihuela O, Ventura MD, Avila-Diaz M, Cisneros A, Vicente-Martinez M, et al. Echocardiographic, electrocardiographic and blood pressure changes induced by icodextrin solution in diabetic patients on peritoneal dialysis. Kidney International Supplement. 2008(108):S125–30.

[68] Mehmet S, Quan G, Thomas S, Goldsmith D. Important causes of hypoglycaemia in patients with diabetes on peritoneal dialysis. Diabetic Medicine: AJournal of the British Diabetic Association. 2001;18(8):679–82.

[69] Woodrow G, Oldroyd B, Stables G, Gibson J, Turney JH, Brownjohn AM. Effects of icodextrin in automated peritoneal dialysis on blood pressure and bioelectrical impedance analysis. Nephrology, Dialysis, Transplantation: Official Publication of the European Dialysis and Transplant Association – European Renal Association. 2000;15(6):862–6.

[70] Ballout A, Garcia-Lopez E, Struyven J, Marechal C, Goffin E. Double-dose icodextrin to increase ultrafiltration in PD patients with inadequate ultrafiltration. Peritoneal Dialysis International: Journal of the International Society for Peritoneal Dialysis. 2011;31(1):91–4.

[71] Dousdampanis P, Trigka K, Chu M, Khan S, Venturoli D, Oreopoulos DG, et al. Two icodextrin exchanges per day in peritoneal dialysis patients with ultrafiltration failure: one center's experience and review of the literature. International Urology and Nephrology. 2011;43(1):203–9.

[72] Gobin J, Fernando S, Santacroce S, Finkelstein FO. The utility of two daytime icodextrin exchanges to reduce dextrose exposure in automated peritoneal dialysis patients: a pilot study of nine patients. Blood Purification. 2008;26(3):279–83.

[73] Sav T, Oymak O, Inanc MT, Dogan A, Tokgoz B, Utas C. Effects of twice-daily icodextrin administration on blood pressure and left ventricular mass in patients on continuous ambulatory peritoneal dialysis. Peritoneal Dialysis International: Journal of the International Society for Peritoneal Dialysis. 2009;29(4):443–9.

[74] Tjiong HL, Swart R, van den Berg JW, Fieren MW. Amino Acid-based peritoneal dialysis solutions for malnutrition: new perspectives. Peritoneal Dialysis International: Journal of the International Society for Peritoneal Dialysis. 2009;29(4):384–93.

[75] Jones M, Hagen T, Boyle CA, Vonesh E, Hamburger R, Charytan C, et al. Treatment of malnutrition with 1.1% amino acid peritoneal dialysis solution: results of a multicenter outpatient study. American Journal of Kidney Diseases: The Official Journal of the National Kidney Foundation. 1998;32(5):761–9.

[76] Li PK, Culleton BF, Ariza A, Do JY, Johnson DW, Sanabria M, et al. Randomized, controlled trial of glucose-sparing peritoneal dialysis in diabetic patients. Journal of the American Society of Nephrology: JASN. 2013;24(11):1889–900.

[77] Mendelson AA, Guan Q, Chafeeva I, da Roza GA, Kizhakkedathu JN, Du C. Hyper-branched polyglycerol is an efficacious and biocompatible novel osmotic agent in a rodent model of peritoneal dialysis. Peritoneal Dialysis International: Journal of the International Society for Peritoneal Dialysis. 2013;33(1):15–27.

[78] Davies S, Carlsson O, Simonsen O, Johansson AC, Venturoli D, Ledebo I, et al. The effects of low-sodium peritoneal dialysis fluids on blood pressure, thirst and volume status. Nephrology, Dialysis, Transplantation: Official Publication of the European Dialysis and Transplant Association – European Renal Association. 2009;24(5):1609–17.

[79] Nakayama M, Kawaguchi Y, Yokoyama K, Kubo H, Miura Y, Watanabe S, et al. Anti-hypertensive effect of low Na connection (120 mEq/l) solution for CAPD patients. Clinical Nephrology. 1994;41(6):357–63.

[80] Nakayama M, Yokoyama K, Kubo H, Matsumoto H, Hasegawa T, Shigematsu T, et al. The effect of ultra-low sodium dialysate in CAPD. A kinetic and clinical analysis. Clinical Nephrology. 1996;45(3):188–93.

[81] Rutkowski B, Tam P, van der Sande FM, Vychytil A, Schwenger V, Himmele R, et al. Low-sodium versus standard-sodium peritoneal dialysis solution in hypertensive patients: arandomized controlled trial. American Journal of Kidney Diseases: The Official Journal of the National Kidney Foundation. 2016;67(5):753–61.

Chapter 3

# Pharmacological Preservation of Peritoneal Membrane in Peritoneal Dialysis

Guadalupe Gónzalez-Mateo, Juan Manuel Gallardo, José Antonio Sánchez-Tomero, Pedro Majano, Elizabeth Flores-Maldonado, Ramón Paniagua, Rafael Selgas, Manuel López-Cabrera and Abelardo Aguilera

Additional information is available at the end of the chapter

http://dx.doi.org/10.5772/64469

**Abstract**

Peritoneal dialysis (PD) is an established renal replacement therapy for renal disease. It is based on the capacity of the peritoneum to act as a semipermeable membrane for the exchange of toxic solutes and water, which is called ultrafiltration capacity. Peritoneal membrane (PM) is lined by a monolayer of mesothelial cells (MCs), which lay on an extracellular matrix bed where other cell types and blood and lymphatic vessels can be found. Long-term exposure to hyperosmotic PD fluids (PDFs), peritonitis or hemoperitoneum causes peritoneal injury by the generation of an inflammatory state. Inflammatory cells and their mediators initiate a cascade of reactions promoting alterations in peritoneal cells, loss of MCs, fibrosis, vasculopathy, and angiogenesis, leading to ultrafiltration failure. Recent studies support that the so-called "mesothelial to mesenchymal transition" process of the MCs runs parallel to the anatomical and functional ridging of PM, which suggests that its inhibition might slow down or stop the PM damage. The fight against PM damage begins with the improvement in PDF biocompatibility. Complementary to this, an alternative approach to preserve the PM might be the use of pharmacological agents or molecular strategies. Here, we explain the existing research models for the development of new therapies and analyze several therapeutic options tested with them.

**Keywords:** biocompatible fluids, mesothelial to mesenchymal transition, peritoneal membrane failure, inflammation, research models, PD solutions low in GDPs, pharmacotherapy

## 1. Introduction

Peritoneal dialysis (PD) is an established form of renal replacement therapy that uses the peritoneal membrane (PM) as a semipermeable barrier for the exchange of toxic substances and water [1, 2]. The use of this technique has increased during the last years [2, 3], possibly due to the technique improvement, especially in terms of peritonitis prevention and biocompatibility of the PD fluids (PDFs). Nowadays, PD rivals with hemodialysis (HD) in terms of morbidity, mortality, adequacy, and water balance [4–6].

Peritonitis and ultrafiltration failure (UFF), with a clinical result of extracellular volume overload and an increased cardiovascular risk, are still the major factors contributing to technique dropouts [2, 7, 8]. The systemic and local complications associated with PD are the challenge of clinical and basic researchers, both with the same aim of improving the long-term preservation of the PM function.

Peritoneal deterioration due to PD (endogenous and exogenous factors) starts with the induction of an inflammatory state, what damages the mesothelial layer and afterwards the whole structure of the PM, compromising its integrity and promoting angiogenesis and fibrosis. These alterations are responsible for the UFF that leads to technique malfunction.

The mesothelial cell (MC) monolayer is the first line of contact between the body and the PDF. The inflammatory process generated, combined with the accumulation of glucose-degradation products (GDPs), advance glycation end-products (AGEs), and others, can trigger a process called mesothelial to mesenchymal transition (MMT) [2, 8]. This process consist in the loss of baso-apical and base-lateral polarity of the MCs, which acquire a fibroblastoid phenotype, invade the submesothelium, and synthesize a large amount of extracellular matrix component (EMC) and pro-angiogenic and lymphatic factors [2]. Therefore, given the role of MMT in the deterioration of the PM, this process can be considered a therapeutic target [9].

Different strategies have been tested *ex vivo*, *in vivo*, and *in vitro* targeting different processes to achieve PM amelioration. This chapter updates the knowledge regarding the processes involved in the deterioration of the PM with specially emphasis on the possibility of using drugs capable of preventing or ameliorating peritoneal damage.

## 2. Understanding peritoneal deterioration: models for research

The three most commonly used methods to study the local and systemic alterations related to PD are the following: the first method is the analysis of cytokines, chemokines, and soluble factors present in PD effluents of patients; the second method is the culture *ex vivo* of cells floating on these effluents (human peritoneal mesothelial cells, from now on called HPMCs; or inflammatory cells) and the use *in vitro* of mesothelial cells extracted from omentum of donors (HOMCs); and the third method is the use of animal models to mimic *in vivo* what happens during the exposition to PD fluids.

Big efforts have been done to achieve *in vivo* animal models, not only to understand the structure and function of the PM but also to resemble PD treatment in human patients, as it is the best way to analyze all the possible elements implicated. With this purpose, several groups have focused on different species, obtaining interesting models where different parameters can be analyzed. Rats and mice are the preferable animal species for these *in vivo* models due to their reduced size, quick metabolism, and easy handling [10].

Along the following sections, we will go deeper on the studies that have been done with these different methods to understand peritoneal deterioration during PD and to develop therapeutic strategies to protect the peritoneum.

## 3. Peritoneal alterations suffered during PD

The PM is lined by a single layer of MCs, which lay on a compact zone of connective tissue that contains few fibroblasts, mast cells, macrophages, and vessels [11, 12]. The PM acts in PD as a permeable barrier across which ultrafiltration and solute diffusion take place.

The long-term exposure to hyperosmotic, hyperglycemic, and low pH of PDFs, as well as repeated episodes of bacterial and fungal infections (acute peritonitis) or hemoperitoneum, induces inflammatory and uncontrolled reparative responses, causing injury to the peritoneum [2, 13–16]. In this scenario, the peritoneum becomes progressively denuded of MCs and undergoes fibrosis and neovascularisation. Such structural alterations are considered the major cause of the loss of the peritoneal dialytic capacity (UFF) [2, 8, 17–19].

### 3.1. Inflammation

The local injury induced by classical glucose-based PD fluids is mediated, at least in part, by the presence of GDPs and by the acidic pH. GDPs through the formation of (AGEs) may stimulate the production of extracellular matrix components (ECMs) as well as the synthesis of profibrotic and angiogenic factors [2, 8]. Both infectious and noninfectious factors activate the immune system orchestrating cellular responses. Inflammatory cells secrete large number of cytokines, growth factors, and chemokines to establish a complex network that feed backs resulting in sustained chronic inflammation, which might trigger the fibrogenic and angiogenic processes associated with the ultrafiltration failure [2, 14, 20–23]. This leads to an increased tendency toward plasma exudations that contain fibrin and coagulation factors. The fibrins in the exudates contribute to the intestinal adhesions and formation of fibrin capsule [19].

### 3.2. Mesothelial to mesenchymal transition (MMT)

MMT is a physiological process necessary for tissue repair. However, in uncontrolled conditions, it is not autoregulated, inducing functional and structural changes in the PM. MMT progression is regulated by complex signaling pathways that can collaborate to accelerate or complete the trans-differentiation: delta-like jagged Notch, receptors for TGF/Smads, integrins, tirosine kinase receptors, inflammation, and hypoxia (**Figure 1**). The list of pathways involved in MMT is in constant growth, and other routes have also been described.

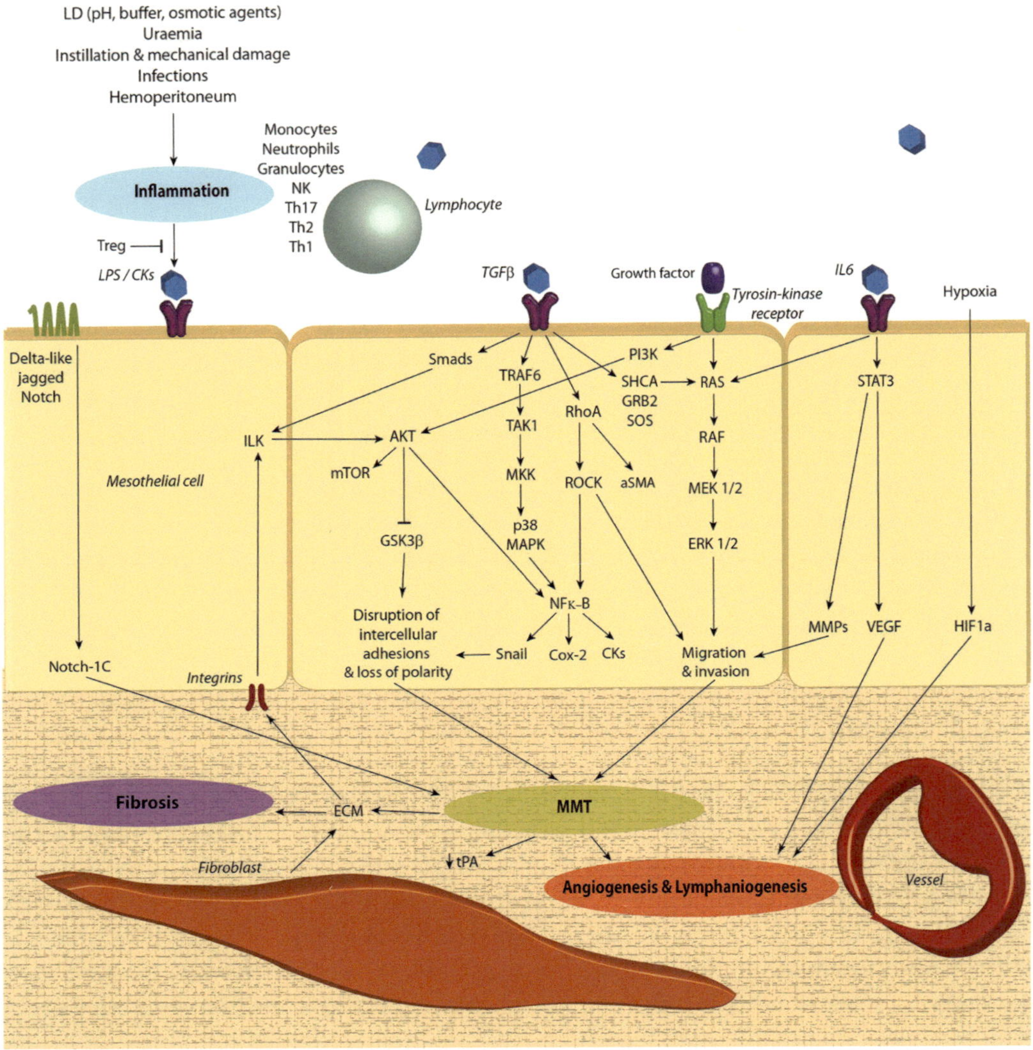


**Figure 1.** Up to day of the molecular networks that regulate MMT. MMT, mesothelial-to-mesenchymal transition; TGFβ, transforming growth factor-β; TGFβR, TGFβ receptor; MMPs, matrix metalloproteinases; GSK3β, glycogen-synthase kinase-3β; ILK, integrin-linked kinase; MAPK, mitogen-activated protein kinase; RAS–RAF–MEK–ERK pathway, extracellular signal-regulated kinases (MEK: Mitogen-activated protein kinase. ERK: extracellular signal–regulated kinase); NF-kB, nuclear factor-kB; PI3K, phosphatidylinositol 3-kinase; TAK1, TGF-beta activated kinase 1; VEGF, vascular endothelial growth factor; ECM, extracellular matrix; mTOR, mammalian TOR; Notch-IC, intracellular fragment of Notch; COX-2, cyclooxygenase 2; CK, cytokines; Th, T-helper lymphocytes; Treg, T regulatory lymphocytes; SHCA, adaptor protein SRC homology 2 domain–containing-transforming A; GRB2, growth factor receptor–bound protein 2; SOS, son of sevenless; HIF-1α, hypoxia-inducible factor-1α; TRAF6, TNF receptor-associated factor 6; a-SMA, alpha smooth muscle actin; AKT, protein kinase B; RhoA, Ras homolog gene family, member A; ROCK, Rho-associated protein kinase; STAT3, signal transducer and activator of transcription 3; t-PA, tissue plasminogen activator; and LPS, lipopolysaccharide.

In Notch and Hedgehog signaling, glioma 1 can induce SNAIL1 expression, and the intracellular domain of Notch can activate SNAIL2 expression, hence downregulating E-cadherin.

The TGFβ/Smads classical pathway is able to activate different routes. One of them starts when the adaptor protein SRC homology 2 domain-containing-transforming A (SHCA) is phosphorilated, creating a docking site for growth factor receptor-bound protein 2 (GRB2) and son of sevenless (SOS), what initiates the RAS-RAF-MEK-ERK MAPK pathway. The p38 MAPK and JNK activation, another TGFβ-induced route, results from the association of TNF receptor-associated factor 6 (TRAF6) with the TGFβ receptor complex, which activates TGFβ-activated kinase 1 (TAK1) and, as a result, p38 MAPK and JNK [24] (see abbreviations in **Figure 1**).

The integrin pathway is able to activate the integrin-linked kinase (ILK), inducing the serine/threonine kinase AKT, which inhibits glycogen synthase kinase (GSK)-3β inducing MMT [24].

Several growth factors, such as epidermal growth factor (EGF), fibroblast growth factor (FGF), hepatocyte growth factor (HGF), and vascular endothelial growth factor (VEGF), can induce epithelial-to-mesenchymal transition (EMT), activating receptor tyrosine kinases (RTKs). The RAS-RAF-MEK-ERK MAPK signaling cascade represents a major pathway that is activated by RTKs in response to growth factors. Once activated, ERK1 and ERK2 MAPK pathway cell motility and invasion are activated [24].

During inflammation and cancer, interleukin (IL)-6 can promote EMT through Janus kinase (JAK)-signal transducer and activator of transcription (STAT)3-induced SNAIL1 expression. Hypoxia in the tumor environment can promote EMT through hypoxia-inducible factor (HIF)-1$\alpha$ [24].

Finally, MCs lose their basoapical and basolateral polarity, acquire migratory capacity to synthesize large amounts of extracellular matrix and angiogenesis through increased synthesis of VEGF (**Figure 1**).

In PD, endogenous and exogenous factors can stimulate the immune system and MCs in the peritoneal cavity to induce MMT by different routes.

### *3.2.1. Evidence for the involvement of MMT in PM deterioration*

Transdifferentiation of MCs *in vivo* has been described in the effluent of PD patients since 2013 [25]. The authors described that soon after PD is initiated, peritoneal MCs showed a progressive loss of epithelial phenotype and acquired myofibroblast characteristics [25]. Effluent-derived MCs can be easily isolated from PD patients using standard methods [25, 26]. It was described that *ex vivo* cultures of effluent-derived MCs showed two main morphologies: epithelioid and nonepithelioid (fibroblast-like). After analyzing several hundred MC cultures with growth capacity, it could be determined that the frequencies of the different effluent-derived MC cultures were approximately 53% for epithelioid phenotype and 44% for nonepithelioid MCs. The prevalence of nonepithelioid MC cultures appeared to be associated with the time the patients have been subjected to PD and with the episodes of acute or recurrent peritonitis or hemoperitoneum [25, 26]. A less frequent cell culture type (less than 6%) with mixed morphologies has also been described [25, 26]. In the course of practicing *ex vivo* cultures of effluent-derived cells, hypertrophic cells can also be observed occasionally in hypertrophic MCs.

However, the most important evidence of the presence of MMT in both surface and deep (submesothelial) areas comes from studies in peritoneal biopsies of PD patients [27]. The number of transdifferentiated MCs showed a direct correlation with the loss of ultrafiltration, the thickness of the PM, and angiogenesis [27]. Experimentally, it has also been found a positive correlation between the degree of MMT and time in PD [28].

### 3.3. Peritoneal fibrosis in PD, sclerosis, and EPS

Peritoneal fibrosis (or sclerosis) consists on the deposit of ECM proteins (collagen I, III, V, VI, fibronectin, tenascin) in the interstitium, with increased number of fibroblasts (some of them presenting myofibroblastic characteristics) and inflammatory cell infiltration. Moreover, it is usual to find extracellular accumulation of collagen IV and laminin in the basement membrane, and also proteoglycans, polysaccharides, and glycoproteins [18, 28–31].

Peritoneal fibrosis is a term that includes a wide spectrum of structural alterations, ranging from mild inflammation to severe sclerosing peritonitis and EPS, its most serious and dangerous manifestation [31]. Simple sclerosis (SS), an intermediate stage of peritoneal fibrosis, is the most common lesion found in patients after few months on PD and may represent the beginning of sclerosing peritonitis (SP) [30]. The peritoneal thickness is the most commonly used criteria for differential diagnosis. The normal thickness of human peritoneum is 20 μm [19], but after a few months on PD, it may reach up to 40 μm (SS). The SP is a progressive sclerosis characterized by a dramatic thickening of the peritoneum (up to 4000 μm), accompanied by inflammatory infiltrate, calcification, angiogenesis, and vasodilatation of blood and lymphatic vessels [31, 32].

Fortunately, the frequency of EPS is low (0.5–4.3 cases per 1000 patients per year) [30, 31]. However, its severity and the lack of adequate and proved therapeutic options deserve special attention. The SPS is considered as reversible condition, while EPS still progresses even after the interruption of PD treatment [32] and is characterized by a progressive intra-abdominal inflammatory process that results in bridles and severe fibrous tissue formation, which cover and constrict the viscera leading to obstruction of the intestinal tract.

#### *3.3.1. MMT as initial step for SPS and EPS*

Although the pathways to reach EPS from SPS have not been fully established, emerging evidences have indicated that MMT is persistently present in initial and end stages of peritoneal fibrosis [27, 28, 33]. It is not difficult to argue that the MMT leads to peritoneal fibrosis, but the EPS jump is still much discussed [34]. An interesting point is that almost 100% of patients in PD show peritoneal fibrosis or sclerosis, while less than 5% reaches EPS [31, 35, 36], suggesting the presence of another factor that sets the point of no return (**Figure 2**). This factor might be a genetic factor [36, 37]. Different research studies have shown in both, animal models and patients, the presence of MMT in the submesothelium from the early stages to the later stages of PD [27, 28, 31]. Moreover, the amount of MMT was closely related to the severity of the damage and anatomical abnormalities in the peritoneal transport.

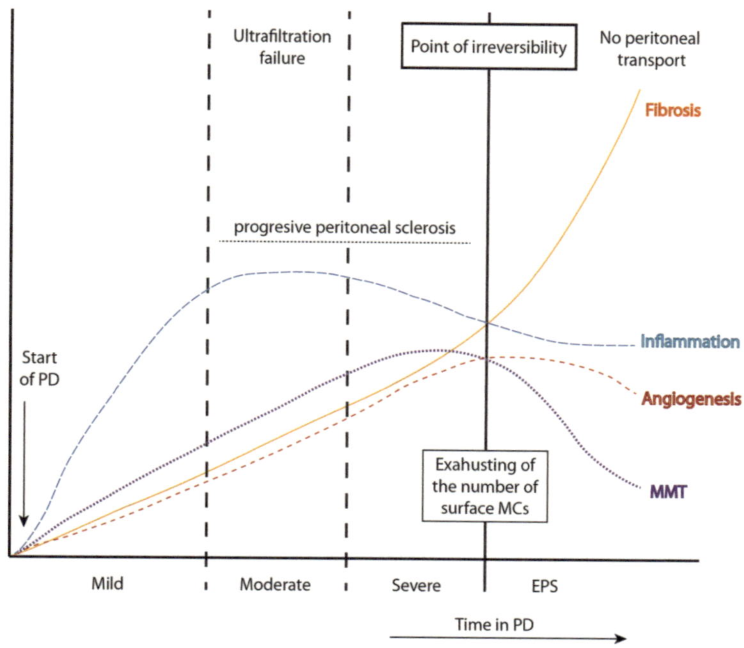


**Figure 2.** Natural history of morphological and functional changes of the PM in PD.

There are several clinic limitations to perform a peritoneal biopsy study in PD patients looking for traces of MMT through time in PD. Another limitation is that we do not have a realistic model of EPS in vivo. Models of EPS developed through Chlorhexidine exposition [38] do not resemble the natural scene lived by the patients in PD.

Accepting that the MMT is an initial step in the peritoneal deterioration process, we must know the mechanisms governing this process. MMT is a generally reversible process that starts with the disruption of intercellular junctions and loss of polarity, followed by increased migratory, invasive, and fibrogenic capacities. The aim of this process is to heal wounds by promoting the recovery of ancestor capabilities of epithelial cells such as cell migration, production of ECM, and induction of angiogenesis [25, 27].

As a patient begins the PD, the PM starts a deterioration process characterized by peritoneal thickening (fibrosis) and angiogenesis. After a variable time period in PD, the PM develops a PM thickening, which can show a moderate or severe fibrosis degree, and type-I PM UF failure starts. These changes occur in parallel with the induction of MMT, resulting in increased number of transdifferentiated MCs in submesothelium as well as other fibroblastic-like cells derived from bone marrow (CD34+) and Endo-MT. Consequently, the number of MCs monolayer is exhausted, and the peritoneal tissue may initiate an automatic, progressive, and irreversible process characterized by severe fibrosis, angiogenesis, and peritoneal adhesion formation: EPS.

### 3.4. Angiogenesis and lymphangiogenesis

Angiogenesis and lymphangiogenesis are phenomena associated with inflammation, MMT, and peritoneal fibrosis. Their relationship is mediated by the production of all VEGF isoforms: VEGF-A is one of the major inducers of angiogenesis, whereas VEGF-C and D of lymphatic vessels [39, 40]. Transdifferentiated MCs are high producers of VEGF, and its levels in effluent and supernatant showed a positive correlation with water and solute peritoneal transport failure. Rapamycin, an mTOR inhibitor, was able to decrease the angiogenesis and specially lymphangiogenesis, maintaining the peritoneal transport in a mice model [41].

## 4. The search for the Holy Grail: more biocompatible fluids, less deterioration

The so-called "conventional" PD fluids (PDFs) are assumed to be incompatible due to the presence of an acidic pH with glucose as the osmotic agent which, after heat sterilization or extended storage, leads to the formation of extended storage, leads to the formation of GDPs (GDPs). These GDPs themselves act as a wide range of cells inducing inflammatory, angiogenic, and apoptosis processes [42–44], but they also collaborate in the formation of advanced glycation end products (AGEs) and definitely accelerate the PM deterioration [45]. In fact, RAGE (AGE receptor) also plays a pivotal role in inflammation, angiogenesis, and fibrosis of the PM [46]. Moreover, it has been demonstrated that single exposure of MCs to GDPs yields AGEs and a proinflammatory response [42]. Interestingly, the relevance and toxicity of GDPs have been demonstrated to be independent from those of glucose. Igaki et al., demonstrated that the GDP 3-deoxyglucosone (3-DG), and not glucose, accelerates the advanced stage of protein glycation [47].

This knowledge has prompted the search of more biocompatible PD solutions free of GDPs and not-forming AGEs.

Wieslander et al., suggested that separation of the dextrose and buffer components during heat sterilization or storage, could reduce GDP formation [48, 49]. This hypothesis was confirmed later in different studies [50–52]. Kjellstrand et al. demonstrated that a sterilization process at an optimal pH (approximately 3) minimizes GDP formation in glucose-containing fluids [53]. Meanwhile, Erixon et al. confirmed that sterilization of glucose at a pH ranging from 2 to 2.6 reduces levels of several GDPs, such as 3-DG, 5-hydroxymethylfuraldehyde (5-HMF), and 3,4-dideoxyglucosone-3-ene (3,4-DGE) [54]. Moreover, storage of the dextrose component at a pH below 4.0 has been shown to substantially reduce GDP formation [55].

Nowadays, different PDFs have been developed, and their use has been widespread in different countries. Many investigations have been developed to discover new osmotic agents to substitute glucose with the finality of avoiding the formation of GDPs and AGEs. Even the glucose-containing PDFs of new generation are now more biocompatible, thanks to the fact that they are prepared as bags with separated chambers that allow the sterilization and storage of the glucose at a low pH, mixing them at the very moment of the instillation in the patient's body. The beneficial effects on peritoneal status are amply documented [56].

In this line, it is important to analyze the impact that the different options of PDFs have on the peritoneal damage related to PD treatment. As commented before, chronic PDF exposition leads to inflammation, phenotype alteration with mesenchymal transition of different cell types (bone marrow-derived mesothelial and endothelial cells), angiogenesis, fibrosis, ultrafiltration failure, and in some cases EPS development. The evidences found *ex vivo, in vitro* and *in vivo* with both animal models and human patients in the most commonly used PDFs nowadays are discussed later.

### 4.1. Glucose as the osmotic agent

#### *4.1.1. Lactate alone-buffered fluids*

StaySafe from Fresenius Medical Care and Dianeal from Baxter are the so-called "conventional PDFs," and they are prepared on a single-chamber PD bag, therefore, presenting a higher amount of GDPs. Balance and Gambro (Fresenius Medical Care) are developed with a double-chamber bag to permit a lower formation of GDPs (although still presence).

#### *4.1.2. Bicarbonate-buffered fluids*

Bicavera from Fresenius Medical Care is buffered with bicarbonate alone, while Physioneal from Baxter is formulated with a mix of lactate and bicarbonate as buffers.

Effluent MCs grown *ex vivo* from patients treated with bicarbonate/low-GDP BicaVera fluid showed a tendency to maintain an epithelial phenotype, with lower production of pro-inflammatory cytokines and chemokines than was seen with MCs from patients treated with a lactate-buffered conventional PDF [57].

In an *in vitro* study conducted by Grossin et al., HOMCs exposure to BicaVera resulted in higher cell proliferation compared to lactate-buffered PDFs such as Balance and StaySafe (at the same glucose concentration), due to their higher viability (as oncosis was demonstrated to be significantly lower). BicaVera, containing lower amounts of GDPs, stimulated less AGE formation and VEGF production than Balance or StaySafe. No effect of lactate on TGFβ expression related to potential polyol pathway stimulation could be demonstrated [58].

Bicavera also showed decreased PM inflammation and fibrosis compared with a conventional PDF (StaySafe) in an *in vivo* mice model [59].

Meanwhile, Physioneal has also showed improved results in terms of PM preservation comparing to conventional PDFs. *Ex vivo*, PDF-induced VEGF, and procollagen III N-terminal peptide (PIIINP) secretion were more prominent in the conventional PDF Dianeal and less prominent in Physioneal. This study also shows that high glucose plays an important role in VEGF secretion comparing to low glucose concentrations, and that GDPs may play important roles in VEGF production by HPMC. Moreover, glucose above 50 mmol/L increased TGFβ1 expression in HPMC [43].

*In vivo*, newly formed vessels and total number of transmigrated neutrophils were higher in Dianeal-treated rats than in Physioneal-treated rats [60].

A recent study from Kumar et al. suggests that glucose-based PDFs may increase the risk and severity of *Staphylococcus aureus* peritonitis, a serious complication for chronic PD patients, as these fluids showed inhibited complement host defenses [61]. For this reason and the fact that it is not possible to absolutely eliminate GPD formation in glucose-containing PDFs, the interest of developing other osmotic agents has been raised in recent times.

### 4.2. Amino acids as the osmotic agent

#### *4.2.1. Nutrineal*

Chan et al. compared the effects *ex vivo* on MCs of dialysate obtained from 4-hour dwells with amino acids (AA)-based and glucose-based PDFs and found that ultrastructure and viability of cells were better preserved and cell proliferation less reduced during AA treatment, although IL-6 secretion by cultured MCs increased [62].

In an experimental *in vivo* study, mesothelial damage and vascular changes could be avoided in rabbits when AAs were used instead of glucose as osmotic agent in dialysis solutions [63]. The enhanced biocompatibility of AA-based PDFs is likely based on both the reduction in glucose load, leading to the less formation of GDP and AGE and the more physiological pH of AA.

The use of glucose-free PDFs, especially AA, seems to preserve MC mass and host defense [64]. Martikainer et al. suggested that an activation of systemic and peritoneal inflammation (measured as increased C-reactive protein levels in serum and inflammatory markers such as IL-6 and TNF-$\alpha$ in dialysate) may appear during the use of icodextrin and to a lesser extent during the use of AA [64]. This circumstance could be due to a better cell preservation rate. In fact, Brulez et al. found better preservation of macrophage function during the use of AA than during the use of 2.27% glucose-based solution [65].

### 4.3. Icodextrin as the osmotic agent

Icodextrin (ICO) is a starch-derived, water-soluble, high-molecular weight glucose polymer (dextrin) that is used as a colloid osmotic agent. Its mean molecular weight is 16,800 Da, and water transport occurs because of the difference in colloidal osmotic pressure. ICO is slowly absorbed into the circulation, and ultrafiltration can be obtained even in a long-term dwell [66].

Currently, very scarce information on the effect of long-term ICO use on the PM is available. In favor of icodextrin, omentum-derived human peritoneal MCs cultured with Icodextrin grew and proliferated adequately [67], and this osmotic agent did not induce upregulation of Snail or Cox-2 as did the PD solution rich in GDPs [59]. Unpublished data by Gallardo et al. using a technique called trans-epithelial electrical resistance (TEER) found that Icodextrin had lower water intercellular transport resistance than dextrose (4.25%) in the MDCK cell line monolayer (**Figure 3**). TEER is an easily quantifiable method to measure the intercellular tight junctions and is a marker of health of monolayer cells. As commented before, the MC monolayer is the first barrier exposed and affected by PDFs, and it can also be used as a marker of solute and water peritoneal transport [68].

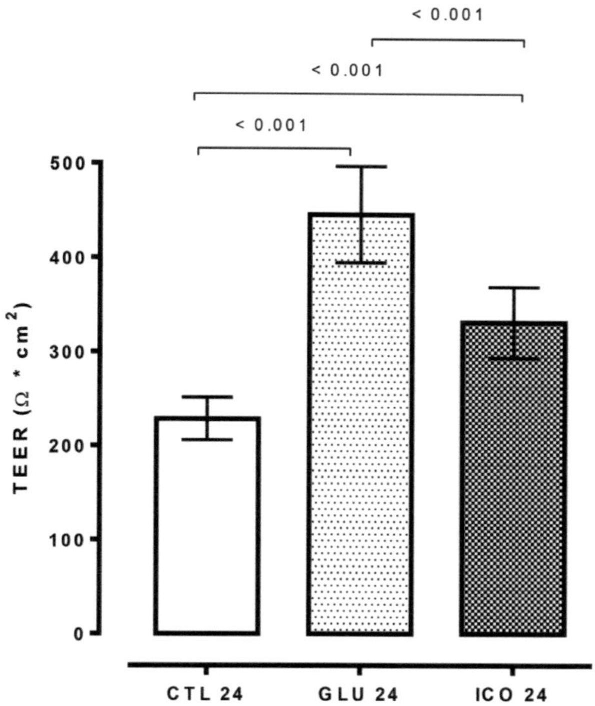


**Figure 3.** Applications of trans-epithelial electrical resistance (TEER) in the measurement of cellular health and PD solution biocompatibility. Results are expressed as ohms per square centimeter [74, 75]. Columns in the figure express means ± standard deviations.

Clinically, Paniagua et al. suggested that ICO treatment is superior to dextrose treatment, allowing a better metabolic control and improved extracellular fluid volume control in diabetic patients in PD [69].

The positive effects of Icodextrin also include improvement in the atherogenic lipoprotein profile, fasting glucemia, insulin resistance, and hypertension [66]. Icodextrin also improves the viability of the PM as demonstrated by Davis et al. [70].

However, because PD uses the biologic membrane as a dialytic membrane, impairment of the peritoneum by exposure to PDF is inevitable, and Icodextrin has also shown negative effects on the PM. This osmotic agent has been related to an induced peritoneal inflammation, increased peritoneal permeability and levels of IL-6 and other inflammatory molecules in effluent. The reaction was transient, but long-term exposure to Icodextrin may irreversibly change peritoneal morphology [71, 72].

Other side effects related to the use of ICO such as allergic skin reactions and aseptic peritonitis have been reported [73].

TEER changes were analysed in MDCK cell monolayers cultured during 24 hours with PD solutions, dextrose 4.24% (GLU 24), and icodextrin 7.5% (ICO 24), compared with control (CTL). Dextrose increased the TEER more than icodextrin, What is associated with upregulation of intercellular tight junction-related molecules. This phenomenon may be related to loss of peritoneal transport capacity at long-medium term in peritoneal dialysis patients.

MDCK-II cultures were obtained from the American Type Culture Collection (MDCK, CCL-34) and maintained in DMEM supplemented (CDMEM) with 10% bovine serum and 10,000 U/mg/ml of penicillin/streptomycin. Cells were harvested with trypsin EDTA, cultured on Transwell permeable supports at approximately 2 × 105 cells/cm$^2$ (Corning Costar), and maintained for 3 days in CDMEM. The concentration of serum was complemented with PDFs, glucose (GLU), or icodextrin (ICO), the last 24 hours before TEER measures. The medium for MDCK cell control was CDMEM alone. The degree of tight junctions permeability to ionic solutes was assessed by measuring the TEER of the cells grown on Transwell permeable supports using an EVOM (Epithelial Volt Hom Meter; World Precision Instruments). TEER was measured before and after PDF exposition. Final values were obtained by subtracting the resistance of the bathing solution and an empty support.

## 5. The new hope: pharmacological interventions to treat and prevent peritoneal damage

As a completely biocompatible PDF will be difficult to achieve, glucose-based PDFs are still needed, and more biocompatible PDFs are expensive, using drugs is a valuable alternative [76]. An advantage of drugs is that they might be administered orally or intraperitoneally, but most of the experiments developed till now are performed in animal models. The challenge for future years is to demonstrate through clinical trials if results in animals are reproducible in humans. New research studies on this line should preferably focus on the potential benefits for the peritoneum of drugs that may serve multiple purposes for PD patients [76].

PD treatment-associated damage can be induced by different factors such as hemoperitoneum, peritonitis episodes, mechanical injury due to the infusion process or the distension of the tissue, and the bioincompatible composition of the PDF, with a nonphysiological pH and osmotic agents that generate an inflammatory response (glucose, GDPs, and AGEs). More biocompatible fluids (low GDP solutions) reduce the peritoneal impact of the treatment but do not solve the problem completely. As the first line of contact between the body and the PDF, MCs are a key target for pharmacological actions. Some drugs have demonstrated the capacity to reduce MMT, such as BMP7, Tamoxifen, TAK1 inhibitors, and Vitamin D receptor activators, among others.

On the other hand, MCs might suffer a mesenchymal transition. Endothelial and bone marrow-derived cells also contribute to the generation of cells with fibroblastoid phenotype [77]. The migratory capacity of transdifferentiated cells can be diminished using anti-VEGF or NRP1 antibodies, as well as with drugs like Tamoxifen. Moreover, it is possible to reduce the increased fibrinolytic capacity of these cells with Tamoxifen, Nebivolol, and heparin.

Other pathologic effects in the peritoneum related to PD are fibrosis, angiogenesis, and lymphangiogenesis. There are an increasing number of drugs able to act against different processes at the same time, ameliorating peritoneal damage and protecting from PM failure.

### 5.1. Immunomodulatory strategies

#### *5.1.1. COX-2 inhibition*

An *ex vivo* study with MCs drained from peritoneal effluent revealed that nonepithelioid cells (that had undergone MMT) express higher levels of COX-2 than epithelioid MCs. The mass transfer coefficient for creatinine, an indicator of UF capacity, correlated with MC phenotype and with COX-2 levels. Although COX-2 was shown to be upregulated during MMT of MCs, COX-2 inhibition was not able to prevent MMT *in vitro*. In mice and rats *in vivo* models of PD, COX-2 inhibition with orally administered Celecoxib decreased peritoneal inflammation, angiogenesis, and fibrosis and preserved PM function [59, 78].

#### *5.1.2. Modulating specifically Th17/T regulatory responses*

It has been recently shown that Th17-mediated and, more specifically, IL-17-mediated inflammatory responses play an important role in PM damage [79]. In fact, pharmacologic treatments modulating Th17 response and/or enhancing regulatory T-cell response ameliorated peritoneal fibrosis and preserved PM function.

Peroxisome-proliferator activated receptor (PPAR)-$\gamma$ agonist Rosiglitazone was shown to protect PM from PDF damage (diminishing the accumulation of AGEs, preserving the mesothelium, decreasing the number of invading MCs, reducing fibrosis and angiogenesis, and improving peritoneal function in an *in vivo* mice model). This effect was associated with augmented levels of the anti-inflammatory cytokine IL-10 (T regulatory-associated cytokine) and increased recruitment of regulatory T cells [80]. Other protective mechanism was the inhibition of Th17 differentiation through a Stat3 cascade blockade, which results in a down-regulation of ROR$\gamma$t and a decrease in IL-17 production [81]. However, the side effects of rosiglitazone have limited its use around the world [82]. New PPAR modulating agents could be promising.

Meanwhile, the activation of immunological regulatory mechanisms by vitamin D receptor (VDR) signaling could also prevent or reduce fibrosis, as observed in an *in vivo* mice model of peritoneal exposure to PDF with Paricalcitol, a VDR activator. The treatment reduced peritoneal IL-17 levels and increased the presence of T cells with a regulatory phenotype, which strongly correlated with a significantly lower peritoneal fibrotic response [83].

It has been recently demonstrated that the leukocyte antigen CD69 controls fibrosis by regulating Th17 response, so it represents a new, yet unexplored, therapeutic target [84].

## 5.2. To preserve the mesothelium

### *5.2.1. To restore the cytoprotective stress proteome*

Exposure of MCs to PDFs results in cytoprotective cellular stress responses that counteract with PDF-induced damage. The cellular stress responses may be inadequate in PD due to deficient levels of glutamine, resulting in increased vulnerability against PDF cytotoxicity. Adding pharmacological doses of Alanyl-Glutamine to PDF restored the cytoprotective stress proteome, resulting in improved resistance of MCs to exposure to PDF [85].

### *5.2.2. To act on the TGFβ signaling pathway*

TGFβ was revealed as a master molecule in the pathogenesis of peritoneal damage in a mice PD model [77]. The strategy employed on this study blocked MMT, endo-MT, fibrosis, and angiogenesis. However, TGFβ regulates many immune, inflammatory, and tissue repair functions, so these data should be taken with caution. TGFβ signaling pathways involved in MMT provide more specific strategies for the preservation of peritoneal membrane with fewer side effects (**Figure 4**). In this context, the endogenous factors, such as HGF and BMP-7, have been demonstrated to block MMT *in vitro*. In addition, intraperitoneal administration of these proteins prevented and reverted peritoneal damage in experimental *in vivo* animal models [86–88]. It is important to note that the use of BMP-7 may be difficult in the clinical practice because of its high price and its association with ossification [89]. Likewise, regulating inflammatory factors that activate TGFβ, such as Celecoxib, could be an option.

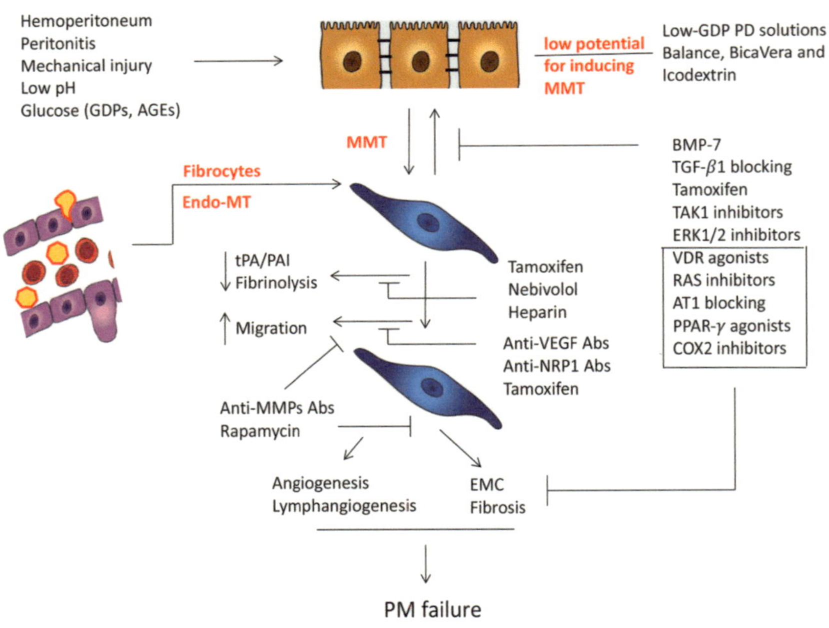


**Figure 4.** Pharmacological amelioration of PD-induced PM damage.

| Agents | Mechanisms | References |
|---|---|---|
| **Anti-fibrotic agents** | | |
| (AcSDKP) Tetrapeptide | TGF-β inhibition | [92] |
| Pentoxifylline | Inhibition of ECM production | [93] |
| Dipyrodamole | Inhibition of TGF-β production | [94] |
| Emodin | Inhibition of ECM production | [95] |
| Simvastatin | Increases fibrinolytic activity | [96] |
| **Anti-angiogenic agents** | | |
| Anecortave acetate | Inhibits VEGF production | [97] |
| Pegaptanib | Inhibits VEGF-VEGFR-binding | [98] |
| anti-VEGFRII | Blocks receptor VEGFRII | [99] |
| TNP-470 | Decreases VEGF expression | [100] |
| **Inhibition of EMT** | | |
| Rho/ROCK-inhibitor (Y-27632) | TGF-β/Samds inhibitors | [101] |
| Antioxidant agent | NF-κB inhibition | [102] |
| Notch inhibitors | Inhibit the induction of snail and repression of VE-cadherin | [103] |
| JNK inhibitors (PS600125) | Inhibition of both ZEB and Rho pathway | [104] |
| CBR1 antagonists | TGF-β/Samds inhibitors | [105] |

AcSDKP, *N*-Acetyl-seryl-aspartyl-lysyl-proline.

**Table 1.** Potential MMT modulators untested in PD.

Other molecular strategies able to block MMT include ILK, RhoA-ROCK, and Akt-mediated signaling cascade inhibitors. These strategies have not been demonstrated yet in PD. **Table 1** shows agents capable of modulating MMT or its deleterious effects that have not yet been tested in association with PD.

## 5.3. Anti-fibrotic agents

Rapamycin, an mTOR inhibitor may diminish IL-17 production. The mTOR activation induces HIF-1 and RORγt and subsequently IL-17 and IL-23 production. Thus, Rapamicin may provide anti-inflammatory and antifibrotic effects and possibly an anti-MMT action, as demonstrated by different groups [106, 107]. Its anti-fibrotic effect is mediated by an increase in arrested MCs and a decrease in MCs dividing DNA [41]. The problem of this drug is the possibility of delayed tissue healing, so its use can be limited to specific moments in the evolution of patients with peritoneal damage.

Other drugs with anti-fibrotic effect include immunosuppressants, simvastatin, pentoxifylline, dipyridamole, diltiacen pyridoxine, tranilast, tamoxifen, statin, and emodin (**Table 1**).

Tamoxifen is a synthetic modulator of the estrogen receptor and is the only agent that has a clinical trial demonstrating its effectiveness in preventing the PM fibrosis or stopping the EPS when it is established [108]. Tamoxifen inhibited MMT in MCs treated with TGFβ in a PD mice model. It significantly reduced PM thickness, angiogenesis, invasion of the compact zone by mesenchymal MCs, improved the fibrinolytic capacity (increasing tPA), and peritoneal function. Tamoxifen also reduced the effluent levels of VEGF and leptin [28].

### 5.4. To act at vascular level

#### *5.4.1. Renin-angiotensin system inhibition*

RAS targeting with intraperitoneal or oral enalapril, valsartan, or lisinopril reduced peritoneal thickening and loss of ultrafiltration induced by 4 weeks of daily hypertonic PDF exposure in rats [109, 110].

#### *5.4.2. Anti-angiogenic and anti-lymphangiogenic agents*

Guba et al. published that Rapamycin decreased the synthesis of VEGF by endothelial cells [111]. *In vivo* exposure to PDF in a mice model, significant reduction in VEGF in PD effluent and in the number of both peritoneal blood and lymph vessels was founded [41].

### 5.5. Anti-fibrinolytic agents

Fibrinolytic capacity of MCs is mediated by a complex balance between pro-fibrinolytic (PAI) and anti-fibrinolytic (tPA, uPA). When fibrinolytic capacity decreases (increased PAI and/or decrease tPA), there is a tendency to peritoneal fibrosis and adhesion MMT as the tPA increases the secretion of HGF [109]. Experimentally, tamoxifen [28], nebivolol [112] and heparin [90] increased fibrinolytic capacity associated with tPA levels increase.

### 5.6. Anti-migration agents

Another way to prevent the deleterious effects of MMT is inhibiting transdifferentiated MC migration. Tamoxifen was demonstrated to inhibit human peritoneal MC migration *in vitro* through inhibition of MMP2 [28]. Although it has not been studied in peritoneal human MCs, anti-MMPs antibodies/peptides are also able to inhibit the cell migration [91].

## 6. Conclusion

Infectious and noninfectious PD-related factors activate the immune system resulting in a sustained inflammatory state that might trigger the structural and functional alterations associated with PD failure, such as MMT, End-MT, fibrosis, angiogenesis, lymphangiogenesis, SPS, and EPS. The methods used nowadays to study the alterations related to PD include the analysis of soluble factors present in the effluents and the use of cultured cells and animal models (which are the best approach to study all the elements implicated). Thanks to the different studies developed in the last decades employing these methods, the challenge of peritoneal amelioration has been deeply studied. New more biocompatible fluids had been shown to improve peritoneal status, but still there is no way to completely avoid peritoneal deterioration, so the use of drugs is a valuable option. Among the different available strategies, immunomodulation and mesothelial preservation presented promising results. Given the connection among MMT, SPS, and EPS, MMT should be considered as a therapeutic target to preserve the PM failure in PD. The use of anti-fibrotic, anti-angiogenic, anti-fibrinolytic, and anti-migratory agents could also represent interesting therapeutic alternatives.

In conclusion, the therapeutic strategies to preserve the peritoneum during PD should aim to improve the biocompatibility of PDFs as well as modulate the inflammation and MMT and their deleterious effects such as fibrosis, angiogenesis, lymphangiogenesis, cell migration, and fibrinolytic capacity alterations.

## Acknowledgements

This work was supported by grant SAF2013-47611R from the Ministerio de Economia y Competitividad and by grant S2010/BMD-2321 (FIBROTEAM Consortium) from Comunidad Autónoma de Madrid to ML-C; from Fondo de Investigaciones Sanitarias (FIS)-FEDER funds, PI 15/00598 Instituto Carlos-III to AA; from FEDER Funds (Fondo Investigaciones Sanitarias ISCIIII PI 15/00120 and REDinREN (RETICS 16/0009/0008) to RS; and CONACYT SSA/IMSS/ISSSTE SALUD 2009–1: 115403 to JMG.

## Author details

Guadalupe Gónzalez-Mateo[1,2*], Juan Manuel Gallardo[3], José Antonio Sánchez-Tomero[4], Pedro Majano[4], Elizabeth Flores-Maldonado[5], Ramón Paniagua[3], Rafael Selgas[1], Manuel López-Cabrera[2] and Abelardo Aguilera[4]

*Address all correspondence to: guadalupe.gonzalez@idipaz.es

1 Research Institute (IdiPaz) & Nephrology Service, Universitary Hospital La Paz, Madrid, Spain

2 Molecular Biology Center Severo Ochoa, CSIC-UAM, Cantoblanco, Madrid, Spain

3 Nephrological Diseases' Medical Research Unit, "Specialities' Hospital," Nacional Medical Center "Siglo XXI," Mexican Institute of Social Secure, Mexico, D.F., Mexico

4 Molecular Biology Unit and Nephrology Service, Universitary Hospital La Princesa, Sanitary Research Institute Princesa (IP), Madrid, Spain

5 Physiology, Biophysic and Neurosciences Department, Research and Advances Studies Center, Nacional Polytechnic Institute, Mexico, D.F., Mexico

## References


[1] Krediet, R.T., *The peritoneal membrane in chronic peritoneal dialysis*. Kidney Int, 1999. 55(1):p. 341–56.

[2] Devuyst, O., P.J. Margetts, and N. Topley, *The pathophysiology of the peritoneal membrane*. J Am Soc Nephrol, 2010. 21(7): p. 1077–85.

[3] Grassmann, A., et al., *ESRD patients in 2004: global overview of patient numbers, treatment modalities and associated trends*. Nephrol Dial Transplant, 2005. 20(12): p. 2587–93. Epub 2005 Oct 4.

[4] Vonesh, E.F., et al., *Mortality studies comparing peritoneal dialysis and hemodialysis: what do they tell us?* Kidney Int Suppl, 2006. (103)10: p. S3–S11.

[5] Collins, A.J., et al., *Mortality risks of peritoneal dialysis and hemodialysis*. Am J Kidney Dis, 1999. 34(6): p. 1065–74.

[6] Schaubel, D.E., H.I. Morrison, and S.S. Fenton, *Comparing mortality rates on CAPD/CCPD and hemodialysis. The Canadian experience: fact or fiction?* Perit Dial Int, 1998. 18(5): p. 478–84.

[7] Selgas, R., et al., *Functional longevity of the human peritoneum: how long is continuous peritoneal dialysis possible? Results of a prospective medium long-term study*. Am J Kidney Dis, 1994. 23(1): p. 64–73.

[8] Margetts, P.J. and P. Bonniaud, *Basic mechanisms and clinical implications of peritoneal fibrosis*. Perit Dial Int, 2003. 23(6): p. 530–41.

[9] Aguilera, A., et al., *Epithelial to mesenchymal transition as a triggering factor of peritoneal membrane fibrosis and angiogenesis in peritoneal dialysis patients*. Curr Opin Investig Drugs, 2005. 6(3): p. 262–8.

[10] González-Mateo G.T., et al., Animal models of peritoneal dialysis: relevance, difficulties, and future. Nefrologia, 2008. 28(Suppl 6):p. 17–22.

[11] Brulez, H.F. and H.A. Verbrugh, *First-line defense mechanisms in the peritoneal cavity during peritoneal dialysis*. Perit Dial Int, 1995. 15(7 Suppl.): p. S24–S33; discussion S33-4.

[12] Di Paolo, N. and G. Sacchi, *Atlas of peritoneal histology*. Perit Dial Int, 2000. 20(Suppl. 3): p. S5–S96.

[13] Garcia-Lopez, E., B. Lindholm, and S. Davies, *An update on peritoneal dialysis solutions*. Nat Rev Nephrol, 2012. 8(4): p. 224–33.

[14] Aroeira, L.S., et al., *Epithelial to mesenchymal transition and peritoneal membrane failure in peritoneal dialysis patients: pathologic significance and potential therapeutic interventions*. J Am Soc Nephrol, 2007. 18(7): p. 2004–13.

[15] Fenton, S.S., et al., *Hemodialysis versus peritoneal dialysis: a comparison of adjusted mortality rates*. Am J Kidney Dis, 1997. 30(3): p. 334–42.

[16] Morgan, L.W., et al., *Glucose degradation products (GDP) retard remesothelialization independently of D-glucose concentration*. Kidney Int, 2003. 64(5): p. 1854–66.

[17] Margetts, P.J. and D.N. Churchill, *Acquired ultrafiltration dysfunction in peritoneal dialysis patients*. J Am Soc Nephrol, 2002. 13(11): p. 2787–94.

[18] Krediet, R.T., B. Lindholm, and B. Rippe, *Pathophysiology of peritoneal membrane failure*. Perit Dial Int, 2000. 20(Suppl. 4): p. S22–S42.

[19] Rubin, J., G.A. Herrera, and D. Collins, *An autopsy study of the peritoneal cavity from patients on continuous ambulatory peritoneal dialysis*. Am J Kidney Dis, 1991. 18(1): p. 97–102.

[20] Topley, N., et al., *Activation of inflammation and leukocyte recruitment into the peritoneal cavity*. Kidney Int Suppl, 1996. 56: p. S17–S21.

[21] Lai, K.N., S.C. Tang, and J.C. Leung, *Mediators of inflammation and fibrosis*. Perit Dial Int, 2007. 27(Suppl. 2): p. S65–S71.

[22] Baroni, G., et al., *Inflammation and the peritoneal membrane: causes and impact on structure and function during peritoneal dialysis*. Mediators Inflamm, 2012. 2012: p. 912595.

[23] Lopez-Cabrera, M., *Mesenchymal conversion of mesothelial cells is a key event in the pathophysiology of the peritoneum during peritoneal dialysis*. Adv Med, 2014. 2014: p. 473134. doi: 10.1155/2014/473134. Epub 2014 Jan 23.

[24] Thiery, J.P. and J.P. Sleeman, *Complex networks orchestrate epithelial-mesenchymal transitions*. Nat Rev Mol Cell Biol, 2006. 7(2): p. 131–42.

[25] Yanez-Mo, M., et al., *Peritoneal dialysis and epithelial-to-mesenchymal transition of mesothelial cells*. N Engl J Med, 2003. 348(5): p. 403–13.

[26] Lopez-Cabrera, M., et al., *Ex vivo analysis of dialysis effluent-derived mesothelial cells as an approach to unveiling the mechanism of peritoneal membrane failure*. Perit Dial Int, 2006. 26(1): p. 26–34.

[27] Del Peso, G., et al., *Epithelial-to-mesenchymal transition of mesothelial cells is an early event during peritoneal dialysis and is associated with high peritoneal transport*. Kidney Int Suppl, 2008. (108)27: p. S26–S33.

[28] Loureiro, J., et al., *Tamoxifen ameliorates peritoneal membrane damage by blocking mesothelial to mesenchymal transition in peritoneal dialysis*. PLoS One, 2013. 8(4)): e61165. doi:10.1371/journal.pone.0061165

[29] Zweers, M.M., et al., *Vascular endothelial growth factor in peritoneal dialysis: a longitudinal follow-up*. J Lab Clin Med, 2001. 137(2): p. 125–32.

[30] Williams, J.D., et al., *Morphologic changes in the peritoneal membrane of patients with renal disease.* J Am Soc Nephrol, 2002. 13(2): p. 470–9.

[31] Di Paolo, N. and G. Garosi, *Peritoneal sclerosis.* J Nephrol, 1999. 12(6): p. 347–61.

[32] Nomoto, Y., et al., *Sclerosing encapsulating peritonitis in patients undergoing continuous ambulatory peritoneal dialysis: a report of the Japanese Sclerosing Encapsulating Peritonitis Study Group.* Am J Kidney Dis, 1996. 28(3): p. 420–7.

[33] Margetts, P.J., et al., *Transient overexpression of TGF-{beta}1 induces epithelial mesenchymal transition in the rodent peritoneum.* J Am Soc Nephrol, 2005. 16(2): p. 425–36. Epub 2004 Dec 8.

[34] Loureiro, J., et al., *Are the mesothelial-to-mesenchymal transition, sclerotic peritonitis syndromes, and encapsulating peritoneal sclerosis part of the same process?* Int J Nephrol, 2013. 2013: p. 263285.

[35] Kawanishi, H. and M. Moriishi, *Epidemiology of encapsulating peritoneal sclerosis in Japan.* Perit Dial Int, 2005. 25(Suppl. 4): p. S14–S18.

[36] Honda, K. and H. Oda, *Pathology of encapsulating peritoneal sclerosis.* Perit Dial Int, 2005. 25(Suppl. 4): p. S19–S29.

[37] Gillerot, G., et al., *Genetic and clinical factors influence the baseline permeability of the peritoneal membrane.* Kidney Int, 2005. 67(6): p. 2477–87.

[38] Lo, W.K., et al., *Sclerosing peritonitis complicating prolonged use of chlorhexidine in alcohol in the connection procedure for continuous ambulatory peritoneal dialysis.* Perit Dial Int, 1991. 11(2): p. 166–72.

[39] Aroeira, L.S., et al., *Mesenchymal conversion of mesothelial cells as a mechanism responsible for high solute transport rate in peritoneal dialysis: role of vascular endothelial growth factor.* Am J Kidney Dis, 2005. 46(5): p. 938–48.

[40] Stavenuiter, A.W., et al., *Angiogenesis in peritoneal dialysis.* Kidney Blood Press Res, 2011. 34(4): p. 245–52. doi: 10.1159/000326953. Epub 2011 Jun 21.

[41] Gonzalez-Mateo, G.T., et al., *Rapamycin protects from type-i peritoneal membrane failure inhibiting the angiogenesis, lymphangiogenesis, and endo-MT.* Biomed Res Int, 2015. vol. 2015, Article ID 989560, 15. oi:10.1155/2015/989560.

[42] Welten, A.G., et al., *Single exposure of mesothelial cells to glucose degradation products (GDPs) yields early advanced glycation end-products (AGEs) and a proinflammatory response.* Perit Dial Int, 2003. 23(3): p. 213–21.

[43] Ha, H., et al., *Effects of peritoneal dialysis solutions on the secretion of growth factors and extracellular matrix proteins by human peritoneal mesothelial cells.* Perit Dial Int, 2002. 22(2): p. 171–7.

[44] Inagi, R., et al., *Glucose degradation product methylglyoxal enhances the production of vascular endothelial growth factor in peritoneal cells: role in the functional and morphological*

*alterations of peritoneal membranes in peritoneal dialysis*. FEBS Lett, 1999. 463(3): p. 260–4.

[45] Himmele, R., et al., *A new neutral-pH low-GDP peritoneal dialysis fluid*. Perit Dial Int, 2012. 32(4): p. 444–52. doi: 10.3747/pdi.2011.00072. Epub 2012 Mar 1.

[46] Schwenger, V., *GDP and AGE receptors: mechanisms of peritoneal damage*. Contrib Nephrol, 2006. 150: p. 77–83.

[47] Igaki, N., et al., *Effects of 3-deoxyglucosone on the Maillard reaction*. Clin Chem, 1990. 36(4): p. 631–4.

[48] Wieslander, A.P., et al., *In vitro biocompatibility of a heat-sterilized, low-toxic, and less acidic fluid for peritoneal dialysis*. Perit Dial Int, 1995. 15(2): p. 158–64.

[49] Wieslander, A., T. Linden, and P. Kjellstrand, *Glucose degradation products in peritoneal dialysis fluids: how they can be avoided*. Perit Dial Int, 2001. 21(Suppl. 3): p. S119–24.

[50] Williams, J.D., et al., *The Euro-balance trial: the effect of a new biocompatible peritoneal dialysis fluid (balance) on the peritoneal membrane*. Kidney Int, 2004. 66(1): p. 408–18.

[51] Passlick-Deetjen, J., et al., *In vitro superiority of dual-chambered peritoneal dialysis solution with possible clinical benefits*. Perit Dial Int, 2001. 21(Suppl. 3): p. S96–101.

[52] Zimmeck, T., et al., *How to reduce 3-deoxyglucosone and acetaldehyde in peritoneal dialysis fluids*. Perit Dial Int, 2002. 22(3): p. 350–6.

[53] Witowski, J., et al., *Glucose degradation products and peritoneal membrane function*. Perit Dial Int, 2001. 21(2): p. 201–5.

[54] Erixon, M., et al., *How to avoid glucose degradation products in peritoneal dialysis fluids*. Perit Dial Int, 2006. 26(4): p. 490–7.

[55] Tauer, A., et al., *In vitro formation of N(epsilon)-(carboxymethyl)lysine and imidazolones under conditions similar to continuous ambulatory peritoneal dialysis*. Biochem Biophys Res Commun, 2001. 280(5): p. 1408–14.

[56] Diaz-Buxo, J.A., *Peritoneal dialysis solutions low in glucose degradation products: clinical experience and outcomes*. Adv Perit Dial, 2007. 23: p. 132–4.

[57] Fernandez-Perpen, A., et al., *Influence of bicarbonate/low-GDP peritoneal dialysis fluid (BicaVera) on in vitro and ex vivo epithelial-to-mesenchymal transition of mesothelial cells*. Perit Dial Int, 2012. 32(3): p. 292–304. doi: 10.3747/pdi.2010.00315. Epub 2012 Jan 3.

[58] Grossin, N., et al., *Improved in vitro biocompatibility of bicarbonate-buffered peritoneal dialysis fluid*. Perit Dial Int, 2006. 26(6): p. 664–70.

[59] Aroeira, L.S., et al., *Cyclooxygenase-2 mediates dialysate-induced alterations of the peritoneal membrane*. J Am Soc Nephrol, 2009. 20(3): p. 582–92.

[60] Schilte, M.N., et al., *Peritoneal dialysis fluid bioincompatibility and new vessel formation promote leukocyte-endothelium interactions in a chronic rat model for peritoneal dialysis.* Microcirculation, 2010. 17(4): p. 271–80. doi: 10.1111/j.1549-8719.2010.00024.x.

[61] Kumar, P.S., et al., *Glucose-based dialysis fluids inhibit innate defense against Staphylococcus aureus.* Mol Immunol, 2015. 67(2 Pt B): p. 575–83. doi: 10.1016/j.molimm.2015.07.017.

[62] Chan, T.M., et al., *Different effects of amino acid-based and glucose-based dialysate from peritoneal dialysis patients on mesothelial cell ultrastructure and function.* Nephrol Dial Transplant, 2003. 18(6): p. 1086–94.

[63] Garosi, G., et al., *Biocompatibility of a peritoneal dialysis solution with amino acids: histological evaluation in the rabbit.* Perit Dial Int, 1998. 18(6): p. 610–9.

[64] Martikainen, T.A., et al., *Glucose-free dialysis solutions: inductors of inflammation or preservers of peritoneal membrane?* Perit Dial Int, 2005. 25(5): p. 453–60.

[65] Brulez, H.F., et al., *Biocompatibility of a 1.1% amino acid-containing peritoneal dialysis fluid compared to a 2.27% glucose-based peritoneal dialysis fluid.* Nephron, 1996. 74(1): p. 26–32.

[66] Konings, C.J., et al., *Influence of icodextrin on plasma and dialysate levels of N(epsilon)-(carboxymethyl)lysine and N(epsilon)-(carboxyethyl)lysine.* Perit Dial Int, 2005. 25(6): p. 591–5.

[67] Bajo, M.A., et al., *Icodextrin effluent leads to a greater proliferation than glucose effluent of human mesothelial cells studied ex vivo.* Perit Dial Int, 2000. 20(6): p. 742–7.

[68] Benson, K., S. Cramer, and H.J. Galla, *Impedance-based cell monitoring: barrier properties and beyond.* Fluids Barriers CNS, 2013. 10(1): p. 5. doi: 10.1186/2045-8118-10-5.

[69] Paniagua, R., et al., *Icodextrin improves metabolic and fluid management in high and highaverage transport diabetic patients.* Perit Dial Int, 2009. 29(4): p. 422–32.

[70] Davies, S.J., et al., *Longitudinal membrane function in functionally anuric patients treated with APD: data from EAPOS on the effects of glucose and icodextrin prescription.* Kidney Int, 2005. 67(4): p. 1609–15.

[71] Alsop, R.M., *History, chemical, and pharmaceutical development of icodextrin.* Perit Dial Int, 1994. 14: p. S5–12.

[72] Martis, L., et al., *Aseptic peritonitis due to peptidoglycan contamination of pharmacopoeia standard dialysis solution.* Lancet, 2005. 365(9459): p. 588–94.

[73] Povlsen, J.V., et al., *Exposure to the peptidoglycan contaminant in icodextrin may cause sensitization of the patient maintained on peritoneal dialysis*: Perit Dial Int, 2003. 23(5): p. 509–10.

[74] Cereijido, M., et al., *Polarized monolayers formed by epithelial cells on a permeable and translucent support.* J Cell Biol, 1978. 77(3): p. 853–80.

[75] Gallardo, J.M., et al., *Tight junctions are sensitive to peptides eliminated in the urine*. J Membr Biol, 2002. 188(1): p. 33–42.

[76] Gonzalez-Mateo, G.T., et al., *Pharmacological modulation of peritoneal injury induced by dialysis fluids: is it an option?* Nephrol Dial Transplant, 2012. 27(2): p. 478–81.

[77] Loureiro, J., et al., *Blocking TGF-beta1 protects the peritoneal membrane from dialysate-induced damage*. J Am Soc Nephrol, 2011. 22(9): p. 1682–95.

[78] Fabbrini, P., et al., *Celecoxib treatment reduces peritoneal fibrosis and angiogenesis and prevents ultrafiltration failure in experimental peritoneal dialysis*. Nephrol Dial Transplant, 2009. 24(12): p. 3669–76. doi: 10.1093/ndt/gfp384. Epub 2009 Aug 7.

[79] Rodrigues-Diez, R., et al., *IL-17A is a novel player in dialysis-induced peritoneal damage*. Kidney Int, 2014 Aug;86(2):303–15.

[80] Sandoval, P., et al., *PPAR-gamma agonist rosiglitazone protects peritoneal membrane from dialysis fluid-induced damage*. Lab Invest, 2010. 90(10): p. 1517–32.

[81] Klotz, L., et al., *The nuclear receptor PPAR gamma selectively inhibits Th17 differentiation in a T cell-intrinsic fashion and suppresses CNS autoimmunity*. J Exp Med, 2009. 206(10): p. 2079–89.

[82] Nissen, S.E. and K. Wolski, *Effect of rosiglitazone on the risk of myocardial infarction and death from cardiovascular causes*. N Engl J Med, 2007. 356(24): p. 2457–71. Epub 2007 May 21.

[83] Gonzalez-Mateo, G., et al., *Paricalcitol reduces peritoneal fibrosis in mice through the activation of regulatory T cells and reduction of IL-17 production*. PLoS One, 2014 Oct, 3. 9(10): e108477. doi:10.1371/journal.pone.0108477.

[84] Liappas, G., et al., *Immune regulatory molecule CD69 controls peritoneal fibrosis*. J Am Soc Nephrol, 2016 May 5. pii: ASN.2015080909. [Epub ahead of print].

[85] Kratochwill, K., et al., *Alanyl-glutamine dipeptide restores the cytoprotective stress proteome of mesothelial cells exposed to peritoneal dialysis fluids*. Nephrol Dial Transplant, 2012. 27(3): p. 937–46.

[86] Yu, M.A., et al., *HGF and BMP-7 ameliorate high glucose-induced epithelial-to-mesenchymal transition of peritoneal mesothelium*. J Am Soc Nephrol, 2009. 20(3): p. 567–81. doi: 10.1681/ASN.2008040424. Epub 2009 Feb 4.

[87] Loureiro, J., et al., *BMP-7 blocks mesenchymal conversion of mesothelial cells and prevents peritoneal damage induced by dialysis fluid exposure*. Nephrol Dial Transplant, 2010. 25(4): p. 1098–108. doi: 10.1093/ndt/gfp618. Epub 2010 Jan 12.

[88] Matsuoka, T., et al., *Hepatocyte growth factor prevents peritoneal fibrosis in an animal model of encapsulating peritoneal sclerosis*. J Nephrol, 2008. 21(1): p. 64–73. Pharmacological Preservation of Peritoneal Membrane in Peritoneal Dialysis 23

[89] Friedlaender, G.E., et al., *Osteogenic protein-1 (bone morphogenetic protein-7) in the treatment of tibial nonunions*. J Bone Joint Surg Am, 2001. 83-A Suppl. 1 (Pt 2): p. S151–8.

[90] Del Peso, G., et al., *Effect of self-administered intraperitoneal bemiparin on peritoneal transport and ultrafiltration capacity in peritoneal dialysis patients with membrane dysfunction. A randomized, multi-centre open clinical trial*. Nephrol Dial Transplant, 2012. 27(5): p. 2051–8.

[91] Dufour, A., et al., *Role of matrix metalloproteinase-9 dimers in cell migration: design of inhibitory peptides*. J Biol Chem, 2010. 285(46): p. 35944–56. doi: 10.1074/jbc.M109.091769. Epub 2010 Sep 13.

[92] Kanasaki, K., et al., *N-acetyl-seryl-aspartyl-lysyl-proline inhibits TGF-beta-mediated plasminogen activator inhibitor-1 expression via inhibition of Smad pathway in human mesangial cells*. J Am Soc Nephrol, 2003. 14(4): p. 863–72.

[93] Fang, C.C., et al., *Pentoxifylline inhibits human peritoneal mesothelial cell growth and collagen synthesis: effects on TGF-beta*. Kidney Int, 2000. 57(6): p. 2626–33.

[94] Hung, K.Y., et al., *Dipyridamole inhibits TGF-beta-induced collagen gene expression in human peritoneal mesothelial cells*. Kidney Int, 2001. 60(4): p. 1249–57.

[95] Chan, T.M., et al., *Emodin ameliorates glucose-induced matrix synthesis in human peritoneal mesothelial cells*. Kidney Int, 2003. 64(2): p. 519–33.

[96] Haslinger, B., et al., *Simvastatin suppresses tissue factor expression and increases fibrinolytic activity in tumor necrosis factor-alpha-activated human peritoneal mesothelial cells*. Kidney Int, 2003. 63(6): p. 2065–74.

[97] Penn, J.S., et al., *The effect of an angiostatic steroid on neovascularization in a rat model of retinopathy of prematurity*. Invest Ophthalmol Vis Sci, 2001. 42(1): p. 283–90.

[98] Vinores, S.A., *Technology evaluation: pegaptanib, Eyetech/Pfizer*. Curr Opin Mol Ther, 2003. 5(6): p. 673–9.

[99] Li, R., et al., *Production of neutralizing monoclonal antibody against human vascular endothelial growth factor receptor II*. Acta Pharmacol Sin, 2004. 25(10): p. 1292–8.

[100] Yoshio, Y., et al., *TNP-470, an angiogenesis inhibitor, suppresses the progression of peritoneal fibrosis in mouse experimental model*. Kidney Int, 2004. 66(4): p. 1677–85.

[101] Nagatoya, K., et al., *Y-27632 prevents tubulointerstitial fibrosis in mouse kidneys with unilateral ureteral obstruction*. Kidney Int, 2002. 61(5): p. 1684–95.

[102] Huber, M.A., et al., *NF-kappaB is essential for epithelial-mesenchymal transition and metastasis in a model of breast cancer progression*. J Clin Invest, 2004. 114(4): p. 569–81.

[103] Timmerman, L.A., et al., *Notch promotes epithelial-mesenchymal transition during cardiac development and oncogenic transformation*. Genes Dev, 2004. 18(1): p. 99–115. Epub 2003 Dec 30.

[104] Das, S., et al., *Complete reversal of epithelial to mesenchymal transition requires inhibition of both ZEB expression and the Rho pathway*. BMC Cell Biol, 2009. 10: p. 94. doi: 10.1186/1471-2121-10-94.

[105] Chen, S.W., et al., *Suppression of CB1 cannabinoid receptor by lentivirus mediated small interfering RNA ameliorates hepatic fibrosis in rats*. PLoS One, 2012. 7(12): p. e50850. doi: 10.1371/journal.pone.0050850. Epub 2012 Dec 12.

[106] Aguilera, A., et al., *Effects of rapamycin on the epithelial-to-mesenchymal transition of human peritoneal mesothelial cells*. Int J Artif Organs, 2005. 28(2): p. 164–9.

[107] Patel, P., et al., *Smad3-dependent and -independent pathways are involved in peritoneal membrane injury*. Kidney Int, 2010. 77(4): p. 319–28.

[108] Korte, M.R., et al., *Tamoxifen is associated with lower mortality of encapsulating peritoneal sclerosis: results of the Dutch Multicentre EPS Study*. Nephrol Dial Transplant, 2011. 26(2): p. 691–7.

[109] Duman, S., et al., *Intraperitoneal enalapril ameliorates morphologic changes induced by hypertonic peritoneal dialysis solutions in rat peritoneum*. Adv Perit Dial, 2004. 20: p. 31–6.

[110] Duman, S., et al., *Does enalapril prevent peritoneal fibrosis induced by hypertonic (3.86%) peritoneal dialysis solution?* Perit Dial Int, 2001. 21(2): p. 219–24.

[111] Liappas, G., et al., *Nebivolol, a β-adrenergic blocker, protects from in vivo peritoneal membrane damage induced during peritoneal dialysis*. Oncotarget, 2016 Apr 18. 7(21): 20133–30146. doi: 10.18632/oncotarget.8780. [Epub ahead of print]PMID: 27102153.

[112] Guba, M., et al., *Rapamycin inhibits primary and metastatic tumor growth by antiangiogenesis: involvement of vascular endothelial growth factor*. Nat Med, 2002. 8(2): p. 128–35.

# Chapter 4

# Peritoneal Dialysis Catheters

O. Obinwa, J. McLoughlin, D. Kavanagh and C. Wall

Additional information is available at the end of the chapter

http://dx.doi.org/10.5772/64024

**Abstract**

In peritoneal dialysis, a well-functioning catheter is of great importance because a dysfunctional catheter may be associated with exit-site infection, peritonitis, reduced efficiency of dialysis, and overall quality of treatment, representing one of the main barriers to optimal use of peritoneal dialysis. This chapter reviews the literature on indications and contraindications for peritoneal dialysis, peritoneal dialysis catheter design and materials, the techniques of insertion, complications, and method of removal of dialysis catheters.

**Keywords:** peritoneal dialysis, Tenckhoff catheter design, indications, insertion technique, removal, complications

## 1. Introduction

Peritoneal dialysis (PD) is a suitable modality of renal replacement therapy in the setting of end-stage kidney disease. It was first used for the management of end-stage renal disease in 1959 [1]. The use of this modality became widespread, following the introduction of continuous ambulatory peritoneal dialysis. However, like in every aspect of medical care, the use of PD can at times result in harm to the patient [2]. A dysfunctional catheter may be associated with complications such as exit-site infection and peritonitis as well as technique failure. Evidence-based criteria for selection of suitable patients, catheter insertion techniques, and management should be employed, so as to reduce the potential for adverse events and subsequent requirement for transfer to hemodialysis (HD).

## 2. Peritoneal dialysis catheter design and materials

Various shapes, lengths, and sizes of peritoneal dialysis catheters have been described in the literature. Each catheter typically has an intraperitoneal component and an extraperitoneal component (**Figure 1**).

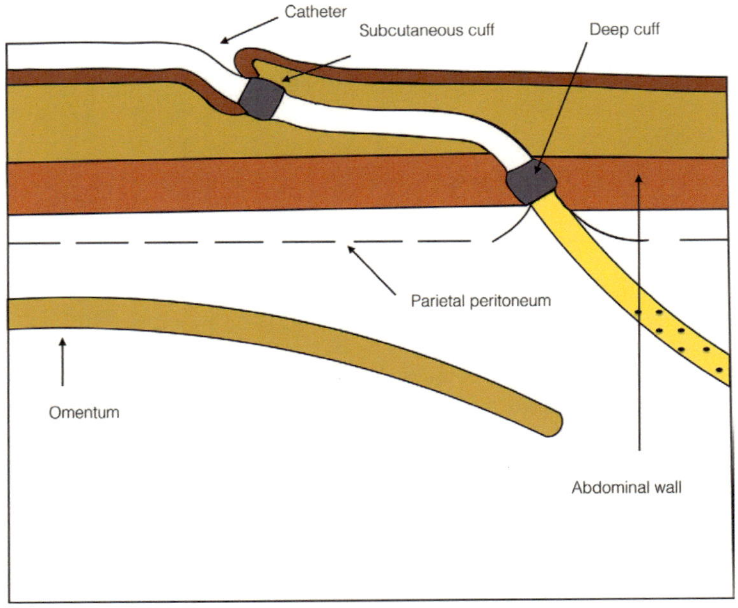


**Figure 1.** Schematic presentation of an indwelling catheter showing the intraperitoneal and extraperitoneal components.

The intraperitoneal component is often a flexible silicone tube with an open-end port and several side holes, which provide optimal drainage of the dialysate. The extraperitoneal component of the catheter has either one or two Dacron cuffs, which permit optimal ingrowth and fixation. A double-cuff catheter is typically used in adults: the proximal cuff is positioned in the preperitoneal space, while the distal cuff is placed in the subcutaneous tissue. The proximal cuff holds the catheter in place, while the distal cuff acts as a barrier to infection. Longer dialysis catheters have also been developed to allow placement of the exit sites in remote places such as the presternal area [3]. Such extended catheters may be useful in obese patients and those with an abdominal stoma.

The choice of catheter used for peritoneal dialysis is clinician-dependent and may be affected by available research evidence. The shape of the intraperitoneal segment may be an important factor when considering complication rates and catheter survival. Typical shapes of catheter tips include straight, pigtail-curled, and swan-neck forms. Although a coiled intraperitoneal segment may minimize infusion and pressure pain, straight catheters have demonstrated significant survival benefits when compared to coiled-tip catheters [4]. Further, surgically placed double-cuffed straight catheters display better survival rates than surgically placed double-cuffed coiled catheters; however, the reason remains unknown [5]. Due to the reasons above, the double-cuffed straight Tenckhoff catheter remains the most widely used catheter in practice. Also, most Tenckhoff catheters have a barium-impregnated radio-opaque stripe, which aids radiological visualization of the catheter.

Further, there has been recent research on the use of antimicrobial modified silicone peritoneal catheters. In vitro challenge tests of these catheters impregnated with rifampicin, trimethoprim, and triclosan showed a long-standing ability for these catheters to kill more than 99% of pathogens commonly associated with PD infections, without the development of significant mutational resistance. These trial results have demonstrated promising results in reducing PD catheter infections. However, human clinical trials have not yet been performed [6].

## 3. Indications and contraindications

There are several advantages of using PD over hemodialysis. The simplicity of use and lower mortality in the first years after starting treatment are the most important.

### 3.1. Indications

Strong indications for PD include obligate situations such as vascular access failure and intolerance to hemodialysis (HD) generally due to cardiovascular instability. Certain medical conditions such as congestive heart failure, prosthetic valvular disease, peripheral vascular disease, and children aged 0–5 years infer a preference to PD over HD.

There are social situations to consider, such as patient preference and living far from an in-center dialysis unit [7]. PD is also beneficial in suitable patients as it facilitates home therapy, increases patient autonomy, and improves the quality of life when compared with in-center hemodialysis [8].

PD has been shown to better prolong residual renal function when compared with HD in patients awaiting renal transplant [9]. Other situations where PD is preferred include bleeding diathesis, multiple myeloma, labile diabetes, chronic infections, age between 6 and 16 years, needle anxiety, and active lifestyle [7].

Peritoneal dialysis has infrequently been utilized for nonrenal indications with variable benefits in conditions such as refractory congestive heart failure [10, 11], hepatic failure [12], hypothermia [13], hyponatremia, dialysis-associated ascites, drug poisonings, pancreatitis [14], and inherited enzyme deficiencies.

### 3.2. Contraindications

One absolute contraindication is the inability of a patient or caregiver to safely and efficiently use the PD catheter and equipment to carry out peritoneal dialysis. Other absolute contraindications include patients with documented Type II ultrafiltration failure (UF), severe inflammatory bowel disease, active acute diverticulitis, abdominal abscess, active ischemic bowel disease [15], severe active psychotic disorder, marked intellectual disability, and in women, starting dialysis in the third trimester of pregnancy [7].

Relative contraindications for PD include patients with severe malnutrition, multiple abdominal adhesions, ostomies [16], proteinuria with protein losses of more than 10 g/day, advanced COPD, ascites, presence of a LeVeen or ventriculoperitoneal shunt, upper limb amputation with no help at home, poor hygiene, dementia, and those who are homeless [7]. Situations where PD is not preferred but possible with some special considerations include obesity, severe backache, multiple abdominal surgeries, impaired manual dexterity, blindness, less-than-ideal home situation, and depression [7].

## 4. Insertion technique

In 1968, Henry Tenckhoff developed the indwelling peritoneal catheter, which was placed through an open surgical technique [17]. Since then, additional approaches including laparoscopic, percutaneous Seldinger, peritoneoscopic, and fluoroscopic placement techniques have been described. Both open and laparoscopic approaches to PD insertion are routinely performed under general anesthetic. Although traditionally reserved for patients not fit for general anesthesia, the percutaneous Seldinger technique of PD catheter insertion avoids general anesthesia and is being favored over recent years for use in PD naíve patients without a history of prior abdominal surgery [18]. In one single-center study, equivalent outcomes were reported with no difference regarding catheter survival at 3 months and 1 year, overall peritonitis rate, exit-site leaks, and primary and secondary drainage failure for open versus percutaneous PD catheter insertion techniques in patients without any history of prior abdominal surgery [19]. The implication is that the percutaneous Seldinger technique may also be the frontline approach to younger and healthier patients requiring dialysis in experienced hands and centers. The surgical and laparoscopic techniques still, however, retain their utility, particularly for insertions considered high-risk because of suspected abdominal adhesions or complex underlying anatomy.

Given that the key to successful dialysis is a well-functioning catheter, there are several clinical points, which must be considered before catheter insertion [20]. Careful patient selection, catheter choice, insertion technique, prophylactic antibiotics, and asepsis during the procedure are all important general concepts. Procedures should be performed by an operator with training and expertise in creating peritoneal access [21]. Antibiotic prophylaxis should be based on local guidelines [22]. Specific considerations for PD catheter insertion include the following:

1. The abdominal cavity must be able to store up to 2L of fluid at any one time before PD should be considered [16]. Therefore, attention must be paid to those with significant abdominal adhesions or entering the third trimester of pregnancy as they usually do not have sufficient capacity for dialysate fluid.

2. Patients with hernia, omaphalocele, and gastroschisis, with several mechanical defects of the abdominal wall should have these defects corrected before contemplating peritoneal dialysis. The lack of integrity of their abdominal wall may prevent PD and may cause a fluid leak into the pleural space [16].

3. The use of PD catheters in patients with intra-abdominal vascular grafts and peritoneal shunts may increase the risk of contamination and graft infection [23]. Therefore, a 4-month waiting period between graft insertion and PD catheter insertion has been recommended by the National Kidney Foundation Kidney Disease Outcomes Quality Initiative Guidelines [15].

### 4.1. Open surgical technique [24]

This is the earliest described technique for peritoneal catheter insertion. Here, a 3–5 cm infraumbilical midline incision is made. Then, the subcutaneous layer is dissected down to the sheath of the rectus abdominal muscle. The anterior rectus sheath is opened, and the muscle fibers are separated by blunt dissection. The abdominal cavity is entered following incision of the posterior rectus sheath and peritoneum. The abdomen is inspected for adhesions, and if any adhesion is present close to the abdominal wall, they are dissected. Next, the patient is placed in the Trendelenburg position; the catheter is advanced into the peritoneal cavity over a stylet. The cuff is finally positioned in the preperitoneal space on removing the stylet. The peritoneum and posterior and anterior rectus sheaths are closed with absorbable sutures, taking care to prevent catheter obstruction and leakage of dialysate. A tunnel is then created to the preferred exit site, which is usually lateral and caudal to the entrance site below the belt line (**Figure 2**).

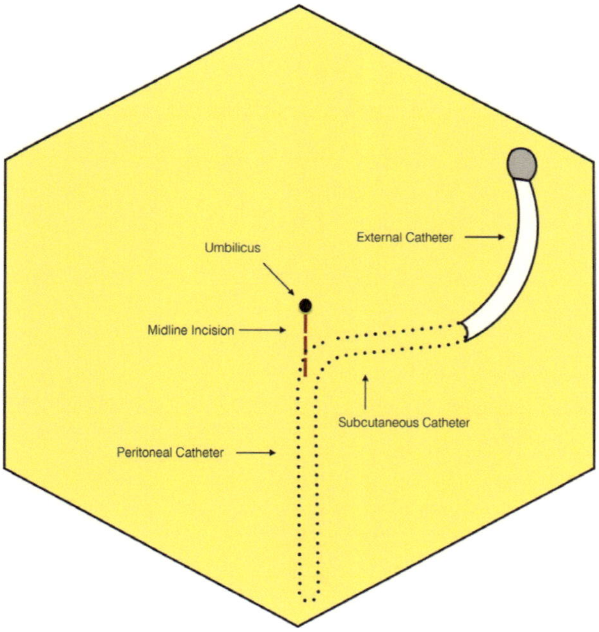


**Figure 2.** Open surgical placement of a peritoneal dialysis catheter. The distal cuff is placed subcutaneously, 2 cm from the exit site. The incision is closed, and the catheter is tested by filling the abdomen with 100 ml of sterile saline. It is important to check for leakage at the entrace site. The drained saline is also inspected to ensure no intraperitoneal bleeding or fecal contamination.

### 4.2. The laparoscopic technique

The laparoscopic approach to peritoneal dialysis is becoming more popular because of its advantage in facilitating a partial omentectomy or adhesiolysis during the initial catheter placement. Approximately 80% of patients who have had previous abdominal operations have adhesions between the omentum and abdominal wall, with 20% having involvement of the small intestine [25]. The laparoscopic PD catheter insertion technique has also been found to be superior to the conventional open technique. This superiority was measured in a higher rate of catheter survival at 1 year and a lower rate of catheter migration (1.3–5.4% following laparoscopic insertion compared to between 7.6 and 17.1% with open techniques) [20]. There was no difference noted in the rates of peritonitis or exit-site/tunnel infections between the laparoscopic and open techniques [20].

A safe technique of insertion is described here. First, a pneumoperitoneum is typically established via an open Hasson technique with a 10 mm access port in a subumbilical midline position. Diagnostic laparoscopy is performed with a 0° lens of 10 mm. A 5 mm right iliac fossa (RIF) port is inserted under vision (**Figure 3a**).

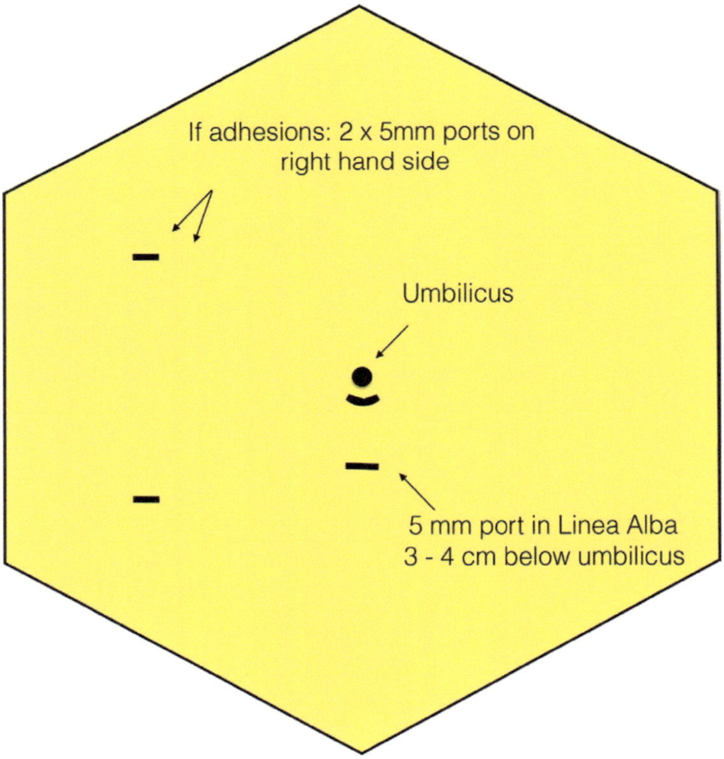


**Figure 3a.** Laparoscopic port placement for PD catheter insertion. If adhesions are present, then an additional 5 mm right upper quadrant trocar is placed into the abdominal cavity, and the adhesions are lysed using instruments via the two right-hand ports. A 5 mm trocar is then placed under direct vision, 3–4 cm below the umbilicus, and the PD catheter is advanced through this port in the linea alba.

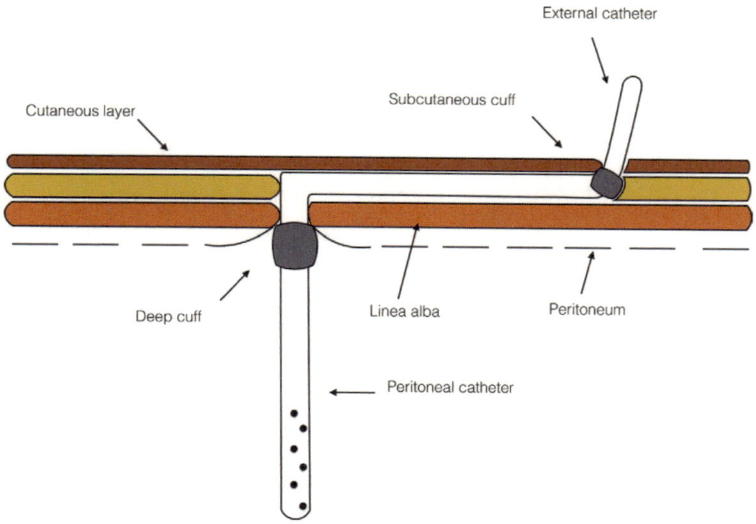


**Figure 3b.** PD catheter insertion through the linea alba. The catheter tip is manipulated into position (Pouch of Douglas in females or behind the urinary bladder in males) using the RIF port instrument. The paraumbilical trocar is removed, and the catheter is then directed to its premarked exit-site location. The catheter is tested before abdominal desuflation. The trocars are removed under vision, and the rectus sheaths and skin are closed.

### 4.3. Percutaneous technique

The percutaneous approach provides a less invasive approach but conversely has an increased risk of catheter malplacement or bowel injury [24]. These complications largely occur because the procedure employs a blind approach. Errors may be limited by the careful selection of patients or by additional use of image guidance for insertion. A blind technique is considered less safe in very obese patients [18]. Other contraindications to percutaneous catheter insertion include previous open abdominal surgery other than appendectomy or cesarean section, a bleeding tendency, and preexisting hernia requiring simultaneous repair [18]. In a recent review, it was shown that catheter survival was unaffected by placement modality (i.e., percutaneous vs. open) [26]. However, early mechanical complications, including technical failures, are more likely to occur with the percutaneous Seldinger technique [26].

Percutaneous insertion of a PD catheter is carried out as a side-room procedure. The catheter is inserted under local anesthesia, and conscious sedation is managed according to local clinical governance procedures. Premedications may include DF118 (dihydrocodeine) 60 mg, intravenous prophylactic antibiotics, and oral diazepam 10 mg [18]. A small infraumbilical incision is made at the entrance site, usually in the midline. The subcutaneous tissues are divided; the anterior rectus sheath is incised; and the abdominal rectus muscles are separated by blunt dissection. An appropriate-sized needle (18 gauge) is placed into the peritoneal cavity. Proper positioning of the needle is confirmed by filling the peritoneal cavity with air or 500 ml of saline. The absence of pain or resistance with filling suggests proper needle positioning. The catheter is placed in the peritoneal space using the Seldinger technique, with the aid of a 0.035-inch guide wire, a dilator, and a peel-away sheath. Of note, the proximal cuff should be in the preperitoneal position at the end of a successful placement. Tunneling and catheter checks are similar to that described for the open technique. The entrance site only is closed.

An alternative placement technique is to bury the external segment of the catheter in the subcutaneous tissues until such a time that PD is required. The rationale is to prevent colonization of the catheter by skin bacteria and to promote attachment of the cuff to the tissue before exteriorization. Results with this technique have, however, been conflicting. The developers noted a reduction in the rate of peritonitis and colonization of bacterial biofilms in the catheter segments between the two cuffs [27]; however, a randomized controlled trial would be required to confirm these results [28].

Units should have clear and well-documented protocols for perioperative catheter care. It may be feasible to commence PD immediately after placement, but this approach should be limited to those who have an immediate clinical need to commence renal replacement therapy [29]. Ideally, PD should be started between 2 and 3 weeks after placement of the catheter. This approach allows sufficient time for wound healing and securing of the catheter cuff. Following insertion, the catheter is flushed with low-volume dialysate until the effluent is clear. Then the catheter is capped and covered with nonocclusive dressings. It is left undisturbed for 10–14 days with infrequent changes of dressing (such as once or twice a week).

## 5. Complications and management

Peritoneal dialysis-related complications remain a significant cause of morbidity and mortality. It is recommended that all healthcare providers who insert PD catheters in each institution should meet at least once every 12 months to review their PD catheter data [22]. Data collected should include details and management of postoperative complications, infections, dialysate fluid leak, and catheter dysfunction. Audit standards for catheter-related complications include bowel perforation rate of less than 1%, significant hemorrhage of less than 1%, and exit-site infection within 2 weeks of catheter insertion of less than 5% [22]. Other standards include peritonitis within 2 weeks of catheter insertion of less than 5% and limiting the incidence of functional catheter problem requiring interventions to less than 20% of cases [22]. A greater than 80% patency rate of catheters at 1 year (censoring for death and elective modality change) is also recommended [21].

Complications can be classified into early (occurring within 30 days from insertion) and late (occurring after 30 days from insertion) [24].

### 5.1. Early complications

#### *5.1.1. Bowel perforation*

Bowel perforation is a rare complication with an approximate incidence of 1% [24]. It usually occurs during entry into the abdominal cavity. Delayed perforation of the bowel by a PD catheter can also occur, but it is more uncommon [30]. The clinical finding of watery diarrhea on commencement of dialysis raises clinical suspicion. Other findings might include sudden onset of abdominal pain and rigidity on examination. Contrast fluoroscopy, colonoscopy, and CT are recommended for diagnosis. Patients should be treated after confirmation of diagnosis. The treatment of choice in bowel perforation is definitive surgical exploration, repair, and removal of the catheter [24]. In the presence of significant peritoneal contamination, a diversion of stoma may be required [31]. However, there are anecdotal reports of successful management, with the removal of the catheter, antibiotics, parenteral nutrition, and hemodialysis [32]. In one case report, the catheter was successfully removed laparoscopically, and the perforation was closed with endoscopic clips [30].

#### *5.1.2. Bleeding*

The rate of serious bleeding complications related to catheter insertions is low and was associated with anticoagulation in one series [33]. Holding anticoagulation therapy for a minimum of 24 h during the postoperative period should eliminate much of the risk [33]. Coagulation parameters should be obtained and corrected preoperatively. When such bleeding occurs, it is usually at the exit site [24]. Manual pressure or addition of suturing can stop the persistent bleeding [24]. Additionally, the initial effluent drained may be bloody, due to the trauma of insertion, but this would normally clear within a few days [24].

#### *5.1.3. Exit-site infection*

The most common causative organisms include *Staphylococcus epidermidis* and *Staphylococcus aureus* [34]. Other organisms include *Pseudomonas aeruginosa*, gram-negative bacteria, and some nondiphtheria *Corynebacteria* [34]. The presence of nondiphtheria *Corynebacteria* species infection favors consideration for antiseptics to be applied as part of the exit-site management [34]. Once established, exit-site infection may respond to appropriate antibiotic treatment when it is superficial. Deep infection may require drainage, catheter removal, and replacement [35]. An exit-site infection that does not respond to treatment may lead to tunnel infection including abscess formation and to persistent peritonitis, which may require catheter removal and occasionally discontinuation of the peritoneal dialysis.

#### *5.1.4. Outflow failure*

There are multiple distinct causes of outflow failure. These include clots or fibrin deposits within the catheter, catheter malplacements, kinking of the catheter within the subcutaneous tunnel, and development of omental wrap or adhesions in the abdomen [24]. Attempts can be made to clear an obstructed catheter: either forceful irrigation using saline or urokinase can be performed; alternatively, advancement of a stiff guide wire under direct fluoroscopic control can be utilized in an attempt to clear [24]. If there is a kink in the subcutaneous tunnel, then an incision is made directly over the kink, and the catheter is repositioned [24]. Outflow obstruction may also occur from malpositioning of the catheter into the upper abdomen. The position of the catheter may be identified on plain film or under fluoroscopy, with the injection of contrast into the catheter [24]. The catheter may then be repositioned with a stiff guide wire, forceps, or laparoscopically [36].

#### *5.1.5. Leakage of the dialysate*

Dialysate leakage represents a major noninfectious complication of PD and includes any dialysate loss from the peritoneal cavity other than via the lumen of the catheter [37]. This may be identified by the presence of drainage at the exit site or the appearance of a bulge underneath the entrance site. Early leaks, occurring within 30 days of catheter insertion, most often manifest as pericatheter leakage [37]. Late leaks tend to develop more than 30 days after catheter insertion and may present with poor dialysate outflow, subcutaneous edema, weight gain, peripheral or genital edema, hernia, and apparent ultrafiltration failure [37].

Leaks may also occur due to a hernia at the entrance site, trauma, or due to the positioning of the proximal cuff on the rectus muscle. Withholding peritoneal dialysis for several weeks may solve the problem [24]. Management options for dialysate leaks include surgical repair, use of lower dialysate volumes, temporary transfer to hemodialysis, and changing from the continuous ambulatory PD modality to automated PD with a dry day. Delaying PD for 14 days after catheter insertion may prevent early dialysate leaks [37], and initiating PD with low dialysate volumes is recommended as a good practice measure [38].

#### *5.1.6. Peritonitis*

This may occur early and manifests as abdominal pain associated with the cloudy peritoneal fluid [39]. In one prospective randomized study, the use of preoperative single-dose IV vancomycin prophylaxis for permanent PD catheter placement reduces the risk of postoperative peritonitis [40]. Further, single-dose vancomycin was superior to single-dose cefazolin in minimising the risk of postoperative peritonitis [40]. Absence of prophylaxis is associated with a high risk of developing postoperative peritonitis [40].

### **5.2. Late complications**

#### *5.2.1. Cuff extrusion or infection*

This complication may occur when the exit-site catheter is placed directly beneath the belt line or when the superficial cuffs are placed too close to the skin. In any such situations, the catheter should be exchanged and a new exit site selected. The use of modified Tenckhoff catheters such as a swan-neck catheter, Ash catheter, and the T-fluted catheter may reduce this risk of extrusion.

#### *5.2.2. Outflow failure*

Outflow failure that occurs after 30 days is most commonly due to constipation and is best managed with appropriate laxative therapy [24].

#### *5.2.3. Peritonitis*

Peritonitis is a leading cause of switch from PD to HD, in particular, within the first 2 years [41], and it is often the result of contamination with skin bacteria. A study by Davenport et al. [42]

reported the highest incidence organism as coagulase-negative staphylococcus in 77.2% of cases. Other organisms in decreasing order of frequency included gram-negative organisms, *Staphylococcus aureus, Pseudomonas*, and methicillin-resistant *S. aureus*. In that study, the cure rates were higher for those centers that used a combination of intraperitoneal gentamicin and cephalosporins than those centers that used oral-based regimens [42].

The cure rates for PD-associated peritonitis are largely dependent on the infecting organism. Systemic or intraperitoneal antibiotics are administered. Usually, a peritoneal dialysis catheter-related peritonitis resolves with proper antibiotic therapy. If the infection persists, catheter removal and transfer to hemodialysis for 4–6 weeks are sufficient for the resolution of peritonitis [43]. There is a strong association between exit-site infections and subsequent peritonitis, with an increased risk up to 60 days after initial diagnosis [44].

#### *5.2.4. Ultrafiltration failure*

Loss of ultrafiltration (UF) and ability to maintain volume homeostasis is another cause of failure of PD. Prevalence rates of ultrafiltration failure resulting in a switch to HD occur in approximately 1.7–13.7% of cases and increase with time on peritoneal dialysis as well, following recurrent peritonitis episodes [45]. UF failure presents clinically with circulatory volume overload. It is important to first rule out other possible causes of volume overload [46].

#### *5.2.5. Catheter migration*

Catheter migration is a significant complication of PD with the potential to cause PD failure, removal of the catheter, and requirement for transfer to HD therapy. Manipulation under fluoroscopy by a guide wire or Fogarty catheter and catheter exchange may be attempted first. Surgical intervention may, however, be necessary in some cases to restore function. Various catheter designs and insertion techniques have been described to overcome this problem [47]. The dialysate can still be infused when migration occurs, but drainage of the fluid from the peritoneal cavity may be difficult. In some cases, the catheter tip is fixated to prevent migration [48].

## 6. Catheter removal

Refractory peritonitis which is defined as failure of the effluent to clear after 5 days of appropriate antibiotics is best managed by removal of the PD catheter [49]. This follows the ethos of "save the patient not the catheter" [50]. Catheter removal prevents morbidity and mortality associated with refractory peritonitis and importantly protects the peritoneum for future PD. Attempts to manage prolonged peritonitis without catheter removal have been associated with an extended hospital stay, peritoneal membrane damage, and increased risk of fungal peritonitis [39]. The British Renal Association has recommended that following the removal of a catheter in patients with nonconcomitant peritonitis, a new catheter can be inserted into the opposite side of the abdomen, either during the same operation as the removal or at a subsequent date. They also recommend that for patients with simultaneous peritonitis that has failed to clear, a new catheter should not be inserted until for at least 2 weeks following removal [51]. Besides the indication for removal based on infectious complications, noncatheter-related reasons for discontinuation of PD include death, transplantation, recovery of renal function, and transfer to hemodialysis because of ultrafiltration failure, poor clearance, or patient choice [18].

Two techniques of catheter removal are described in the literature: PD pull technique and surgical removal. Each technique has advantages. The main advantages of the pull technique over the surgical technique include the following: a general anesthetic or operation is not required; the procedure takes only a few minutes with quicker patient recovery, allowing little to no interruption to work or home schedule.

### 6.1. PD pull technique

Here, the patient lies on a couch or bed, and the dressing is removed. The exit site is inspected for the presence of an infection. In the absence of an exit-site infection, the PD catheter is extracted by applying firm abdominal pressure around the PD catheter site, while maintaining a firm and steady pull on the catheter with the other hand. The superficial cuff may slide off the skin, but usually both cuffs are left in situ. The cuff may become infected at a later stage, and this serves a limitation to this approach.

### 6.2. Surgical removal

This method of removal is recommended for infected PD exit sites. The procedure is usually performed as a day case and follows standard day surgery protocols including preoperative assessment and consent. A general anesthesia is required, and the procedure takes about 20 min. A small incision is made just below the umbilicus. The catheter and cuff are then removed from the abdominal cavity. The incision is closed using absorbable sutures. A dressing is applied and replaced weekly until the wound is healed.

## 7. Summary

A well-functioning peritoneal dialysis catheter is essential for ongoing effective peritoneal dialysis. In order to optimize its function and patient safety, careful patient selection plays an important role. Catheter insertion is performed using several approaches, including laparoscopic, percutaneous, and open surgical, each with its unique advantages. However, there may be complications following insertion, which may necessitate catheter removal and switch to hemodialysis. A regular audit of outcomes of catheter insertions is recommended.

## Key points

- The success of peritoneal dialysis requires a functional peritoneal dialysis catheter in an appropriately selected and trained patient.

- Peritoneal catheterization should be avoided until the need for regular peritoneal dialysis arises.
- There are several catheter designs available, but the choice is often clinician-dependent.
- Numerous techniques for insertion have been described, including open, laparoscopic, and percutaneous techniques.
- Laparoscopic catheter insertion is becoming more popular. This insertion technique has been reported to have a higher rate of catheter survival and a lower rate of catheter migration when compared to open surgical insertion.
- A percutaneous insertion is an option in patients with end-stage kidney disease and multiple comorbidities as it can be performed under local anesthesia. The trade-off may be a higher incidence of early mechanical complications. Recent studies also show this technique to be a viable frontline approach in patients without any prior abdominal surgery with equivalent outcomes when compared to use of the open approach.
- Reasons for removal of PD catheter include nonresolving peritonitis, fungal peritonitis, ultrafiltration failure, and transplantation. Regular audit of outcomes of catheter insertions is recommended.

## Author details

O. Obinwa[1*], J. McLoughlin[1,2], D. Kavanagh[1] and C. Wall[2]

*Address all correspondence to: obinnaobinwa@rcsi.ie

1 Department of Surgery, The Adelaide and Meath Hospital, Tallaght, Dublin, Ireland

2 Department of Nephrology, The Adelaide and Meath Hospital, Tallaght, Dublin, Ireland

## References

[1] Blagg CR. The early history of dialysis for chronic renal failure in the United States: a view from Seattle. American Journal of Kidney Diseases: The Official Journal of the National Kidney Foundation. 2007;49(3):482–96. DOI:10.1053/j.ajkd.2007.01.017

[2] Bender FH. Avoiding harm in peritoneal dialysis patients. Advances in Chronic Kidney Disease. 2012;19(3):171–8. DOI:10.1053/j.ackd.2012.04.002

[3] Crabtree JH. Extended peritoneal dialysis catheters for upper abdominal wall exit sites. Peritoneal Dialysis International: Journal of the International Society for Peritoneal Dialysis. 2004;24(3):292–4.

[4] Hagen SM, Lafranca JA, IJzermans JN, et al. A systematic review and meta-analysis of the influence of peritoneal dialysis catheter type on complication rate and catheter survival. Kidney International. 2014;85(4):920–32. DOI:10.1038/ki.2013.365

[5] Stylianou KG and Daphnis EK. Selecting the optimal peritoneal dialysis catheter. Kidney International. 2014;85(4):741–3. DOI:10.1038/ki.2013.424

[6] Bayston R, Fisher LE and Weber K. An antimicrobial modified silicone peritoneal catheter with activity against both Gram-positive and Gram-negative bacteria. Biomaterials. 2009;30(18):3167–73. DOI:10.1016/j.biomaterials.2009.02.028

[7] Shetty A and Oreopoulos D. Peritoneal dialysis: its indications and contraindications. Dialysis & Transplantation. 2000;29(2):71–7.

[8] Juergensen E, Wuerth D, Finkelstein SH, et al. Hemodialysis and peritoneal dialysis: patients' assessment of their satisfaction with therapy and the impact of the therapy on their lives. Clinical Journal of the American Society of Nephrology: CJASN. 2006;1(6): 1191–6. DOI:10.2215/CJN.01220406

[9] Tokgoz B. Clinical advantages of peritoneal dialysis. Peritoneal Dialysis International: Journal of the International Society for Peritoneal Dialysis. 2009;29(Suppl. 2):S59–61.

[10] Rubin J and Ball R. Continuous ambulatory peritoneal dialysis as treatment of severe congestive heart failure in the face of chronic renal failure. Report of eight cases. Archives of Internal Medicine. 1986;146(8):1533–5.

[11] Konig PS, Lhotta K, Kronenberg F, et al. CAPD: a successful treatment in patients suffering from therapy-resistant congestive heart failure. Advances in Peritoneal Dialysis. Conference on Peritoneal Dialysis. 1991;7:97–101.

[12] Mactier RA, Dobbie JW and Khanna R. Peritoneal dialysis in fulminant hepatic failure. Peritoneal Dialysis International. 1986;6(4):199–202.

[13] Reuler JB and Parker RA. Peritoneal dialysis in the management of hypothermia. JAMA. 1978;240(21):2289–90.

[14] Mayer AD, McMahon MJ, Corfield AP, et al. Controlled clinical trial of peritoneal lavage for the treatment of severe acute pancreatitis. The New England Journal of Medicine. 1985;312(7):399–404. DOI:10.1056/NEJM198502143120703

[15] DOQI N. Clinical Practice Guidelines for Peritoneal Dialysis Adequacy: update 2000. American Journal of Kidney Diseases: The Official Journal of the National Kidney Foundation. 2001;37(1 Suppl. 1):S65–136.

[16] Haggerty S, Roth S, Walsh D, et al. Guidelines for laparoscopic peritoneal dialysis access surgery. Surgical Endoscopy. 2014;28(11):3016–45. DOI:10.1007/s00464-014-3851-9

[17] Tenckhoff H and Curtis FK. Experience with maintenance peritoneal dialysis in the home. Transactions – American Society for Artificial Internal Organs. 1970;16:90–5.

[18] Medani S, Shantier M, Hussein W, et al. A comparative analysis of percutaneous and open surgical techniques for peritoneal catheter placement. Peritoneal Dialysis International: Journal of the International Society for Peritoneal Dialysis. 2012;32(6): 628–35. DOI:10.3747/pdi.2011.00187

[19] Medani S, Hussein W, Shantier M, et al. Comparison of percutaneous and open surgical techniques for first-time peritoneal dialysis catheter placement in the unbreached peritoneum. Peritoneal Dialysis International: Journal of the International Society for Peritoneal Dialysis. 2015;35(5):576–85. DOI:10.3747/pdi.2013.00003

[20] Hagen SM, Lafranca JA, Steyerberg EW, et al. Laparoscopic versus open peritoneal dialysis catheter insertion: a meta-analysis. PloS One. 2013;8(2):e56351. DOI:10.1371/journal.pone.0056351

[21] Flanigan M and Gokal R. Peritoneal catheters and exit-site practices toward optimum peritoneal access: a review of current developments. Peritoneal Dialysis International: Journal of the International Society for Peritoneal Dialysis. 2005;25(2):132–9.

[22] Figueiredo A, Goh BL, Jenkins S, et al. Clinical practice guidelines for peritoneal access. Peritoneal Dialysis International: Journal of the International Society for Peritoneal Dialysis. 2010;30(4):424–9. DOI:10.3747/pdi.2010.00087

[23] Gulanikar AC, Jindal KK and Hirsch DJ. Is chronic peritoneal dialysis safe in patients with intra-abdominal prosthetic vascular grafts? Nephrology, Dialysis, Transplantation: Official Publication of the European Dialysis and Transplant Association – European Renal Association. 1991;6(3):215–7.

[24] Peppelenbosch A, van Kuijk WH, Bouvy ND, et al. Peritoneal dialysis catheter placement technique and complications. NDT Plus. 2008;1(Suppl. 4):iv23–8. DOI:10.1093/ndtplus/sfn120

[25] Menzies D and Ellis H. Intestinal obstruction from adhesions – how big is the problem? Annals of the Royal College of Surgeons of England. 1990;72(1):60–3.

[26] Park YS, Min SI, Kim DK, et al. The outcomes of percutaneous versus open placement of peritoneal dialysis catheters. World Journal of Surgery. 2014;38(5):1058–64. DOI: 10.1007/s00268-013-2346-5

[27] Moncrief JW, Popovich RP, Dasgupta M, et al. Reduction in peritonitis incidence in continuous ambulatory peritoneal dialysis with a new catheter and implantation technique. Peritoneal Dialysis International: Journal of the International Society for Peritoneal Dialysis. 1993;13(Suppl. 2):S329–31.

[28] Danielsson A, Blohme L, Tranaeus A, et al. A prospective randomized study of the effect of a subcutaneously "buried" peritoneal dialysis catheter technique versus standard technique on the incidence of peritonitis and exit-site infection. Peritoneal Dialysis International: Journal of the International Society for Peritoneal Dialysis. 2002;22(2):211–9.

[29] Ghaffari A. Urgent-start peritoneal dialysis: a quality improvement report. American Journal of Kidney Diseases: The Official Journal of the National Kidney Foundation. 2012;59(3):400–8. DOI:10.1053/j.ajkd.2011.08.034

[30] Baek SK, Bae OS and Jang BK. Endoscopic management of delayed perforation of the rectum caused by a peritoneal dialysis catheter. Surgical Laparoscopy, Endoscopy & Percutaneous Techniques. 2011;21(1):e44–7. DOI:10.1097/SLE.0b013e3182093fb4

[31] Finkle SN. Peritoneal dialysis catheter erosion into bowel: amyloidosis may be a risk factor. Peritoneal Dialysis International: Journal of the International Society for Peritoneal Dialysis. 2005;25(3):296–7.

[32] Grzegorzewska A and Deja A. Conservative treatment of perforation of the transverse colon caused by a catheter for continuous peritoneal dialysis. A case report. Polskie Archiwum Medycyny Wewnetrznej. 1989;81(6):368–72.

[33] Mital S, Fried LF and Piraino B. Bleeding complications associated with peritoneal dialysis catheter insertion. Peritoneal Dialysis International: Journal of the International Society for Peritoneal Dialysis. 2004;24(5):478–80.

[34] Teixido J, Arias N, Tarrats L, et al. The microbial pattern of the catheter exit-site infection in peritoneal dialysis: a non-diphtheria Corynebacteria emergence? Nefrologia: Publicacion Oficial de la Sociedad Espanola Nefrologia. 2007;27(3):350–8.

[35] Thodis E, Passadakis P, Ossareh S, et al. Peritoneal catheter exit-site infections: predisposing factors, prevention and treatment. The International Journal of Artificial Organs. 2003;26(8):698–714.

[36] Savader SJ, Lund G, Scheel PJ, et al. Guide wire directed manipulation of malfunctioning peritoneal dialysis catheters: a critical analysis. Journal of Vascular and Interventional Radiology. 1997;8(6):957–63.

[37] Leblanc M, Ouimet D and Pichette V. Dialysate leaks in peritoneal dialysis. Seminars in Dialysis. 2001;14(1):50–4.

[38] Hassan K, Rubinchik I, Hassan F, et al. Unusual cause of late peritoneal dialysate leakage. Peritoneal Dialysis International: Journal of the International Society for Peritoneal Dialysis. 2012;32(3):360–1. DOI:10.3747/pdi.2011.00044

[39] Li PK, Szeto CC, Piraino B, et al. Peritoneal dialysis-related infections recommendations: 2010 update. Peritoneal Dialysis International: Journal of the International Society for Peritoneal Dialysis. 2010;30(4):393–423. DOI:10.3747/pdi.2010.00049

[40] Gadallah MF, Ramdeen G, Mignone J, et al. Role of preoperative antibiotic prophylaxis in preventing postoperative peritonitis in newly placed peritoneal dialysis catheters. American Journal of Kidney Diseases: The Official Journal of the National Kidney Foundation. 2000;36(5):1014–9. DOI:10.1053/ajkd.2000.19104

[41] Jaar BG, Plantinga LC, Crews DC, et al. Timing, causes, predictors and prognosis of switching from peritoneal dialysis to hemodialysis: a prospective study. BMC Nephrology. 2009;10:3. DOI:10.1186/1471-2369-10-3

[42] Davenport A. Peritonitis remains the major clinical complication of peritoneal dialysis: The London, UK, peritonitis audit 2002–2003. Peritoneal Dialysis International: Journal of the International Society for Peritoneal Dialysis. 2009;29(3):297–302.

[43] Piraino B, Bailie GR, Bernardini J, et al. Peritoneal dialysis-related infections recommendations: 2005 update. Peritoneal Dialysis International: Journal of the International Society for Peritoneal Dialysis. 2005;25(2):107–31.

[44] van Diepen AT, Tomlinson GA and Jassal SV. The association between exit site infection and subsequent peritonitis among peritoneal dialysis patients. Clinical Journal of the American Society of Nephrology. 2012;7(8):1266–71. DOI:10.2215/CJN.00980112

[45] Margetts PJ and Churchill DN. Acquired ultrafiltration dysfunction in peritoneal dialysis patients. Journal of the American Society of Nephrology. 2002;13(11):2787–94.

[46] Teitelbaum I. Ultrafiltration failure in peritoneal dialysis: a pathophysiologic approach. Blood Purification. 2015;39(1–3):70–3. DOI:10.1159/000368972

[47] Scott PD, Bakran A, Pearson R, et al. Peritoneal dialysis access. Prospective randomized trial of 3 different peritoneal catheters—preliminary report. Peritoneal Dialysis International: Journal of the International Society for Peritoneal Dialysis. 1994;14(3): 289–90.

[48] Bay WH, Cerilli GJ, Perrine V, et al. Analysis of a new technique to stabilize the chronic peritoneal dialysis catheter. American Journal of Kidney Diseases: The Official Journal of the National Kidney Foundation. 1983;3(2):133–5.

[49] Choi P, Nemati E, Banerjee A, et al. Peritoneal dialysis catheter removal for acute peritonitis: a retrospective analysis of factors associated with catheter removal and prolonged postoperative hospitalization. American Journal of Kidney Diseases: The Official Journal of the National Kidney Foundation. 2004;43(1):103–11.

[50] Piraino B. Peritoneal dialysis catheter replacement: "save the patient and not the catheter". Seminars in Dialysis. 2003;16(1):72–5.

[51] Gokal R, Ash SR, Helfrich GB, et al. Peritoneal catheters and exit-site practices: toward optimum peritoneal access. Peritoneal Dialysis International: Journal of the International Society for Peritoneal Dialysis. 1993;13(1):29–39.

# Chapter 5

# Assessment of Volume Status in Peritoneal Dialysis Patients

Olga Balafa

Additional information is available at the end of the chapter

http://dx.doi.org/10.5772/64023

**Abstract**

Ideal volume status of patients with end-stage renal disease is one of the main goals of adequate dialysis. Volume overload has been associated with heart failure, left ventricular hypertrophy, and mortality, both in hemodialysis (HD) and peritoneal dialysis (PD) populations. The assessment of normal volume status is traditionally based on clinical parameters such as blood pressure, edema, lung auscultation, and chest X-ray. However, these parameters cannot be trustworthy to direct treatment decisions. Gold standard methods of assessing volume status are mainly isotope dilution analysis techniques. However, these methods are invasive and impractical in clinical routine. A number of handy bedside methods have been developed focusing on objective fluid status assessment, both in HD and PD patients. Bioimpedance techniques can estimate extracellular volume, intracellular volume, and total body water, whereas inferior vena cava diameter measurements, biochemical markers, and lung ultrasound provide information about the intravascular filling state and blood volume. Various studies have used the values of the above-mentioned techniques as tools for determining the overhydration of dialysis patients as well as predictors of mortality. Yet, randomized intervention studies based on these methods with hard end points (like echocardiographic parameters modification) have not been published so far in PD patients.

**Keywords:** bioimpedance, hemodialysis, lung ultrasound, biomarkers, overhydration, mortality

## 1. Introduction

Ideal volume status of patients with end-stage renal disease is one of the main objectives of adequate dialysis. Volume overload has been associated with heart failure, left ventricular hypertrophy, and mortality both in hemodialysis (HD) and peritoneal dialysis (PD) populations [1–5]. One routine clinical way to define volume status is to determine the ideal dry weight of the patients. While dry weight in HD patients has been attempted vigorously to be termed during the last decades [6], such efforts have never been done systematically in PD populations, mainly due to the different nature of the dialysis procedure. Krediet [7] suggested to define optimal volume status as the weight associated with a normal extracellular water/volume (ECV).

| Technique | What is estimated | Advantages | Limitations |
|---|---|---|---|
| Dilution tracers | ECV, TBW | Gold standard method | Invasive, not for everyday clinical practice |
| IVC | Intravascular filling–BV | Correlation with cardiac Function, noninvasive | Experienced cardiologist |
| Bioimpedance | ECV, ICV, TBW | Easy, noninvasive, fluid volumes in liters | No standardization<br>Influenced by hypoalbuminemia and muscle wasting |
| Biomarkers | Intravascular filling–BV | Noninvasive | Wide variability<br>Influenced by cardiac dysfunction |
| Lung ultrasound | Intravascular filling–BV | Noninvasive, easy | No estimation of TBW, ECV<br>Little experience in PD |

IVC, inferior vena cava diameter; ECV, extracellular volume; ICV, intracellular volume; TBW, total body water; BV, blood volume.

**Table 1.** Techniques for assessment of volume status in PD populations.

The assessment of euvolemia—normal volume status—is traditionally based on clinical parameters and examinations such as blood pressure, edema, lung auscultation, and chest X-ray. However, these parameters cannot be reliable to guide treatment decisions. Agarwal et al. [8], in a cross-sectional trial in HD population, showed that pedal edema did not reflect volume status. No study so far has showed a direct relation between clinically assessed fluid overload and outcome in PD patients. Despite the lack of such trials, ISPD guidelines suggest that "hydration status should be assessed clinically on a regular basis during every follow-up visit and more often if clinically indicated" [9].

The clinical aim of defining the ideal volume status is more urgent in PD population, as some trials imply that PD patients are much more volume-overloaded than HD patients [10]. This finding depends on the methods used for assessing volume status; bioimpedance techniques showed that PD patients presented with higher ECV compared with HD patients, even before the hemodialysis session [10, 11], while serum biomarker levels had no differences between them.

Gold standard methods of assessing volume status are mainly isotope dilution analysis techniques. Deuterium and tritium dilution are preferred means to measure total body water (TBW), while bromine chloride and sucrose dilution yield data on ECV [12]. DEXA dual-energy X-ray absorptiometry can provide data about fat mass, lean soft tissue mass, and bone tissue mass [13]. However, these methods are invasive, expensive, and unfeasible in clinical routine.

A number of practical bedside methods have been developed focusing on objective fluid status assessment, both in HD and PD patients. Bioimpedance techniques can estimate ECV, intracellular volume (ICV), and TBW, whereas inferior vena cava diameter measurements, biochemical markers (such as atrial natriuretic peptide, ANP and brain natriuretic peptide, BNP), and lung ultrasound provide information about the intravascular filling state/blood volume (**Table 1**).

## 2. How to assess fluid status

### 2.1. Inferior vena cava diameter

Measurement of the diameter of inferior vena cava (IVC) and its decrease on deep inspiration (collapsibility index—CI) by echocardiography allows an accurate assessment of dry weight in hemodialysis patients. The diameter of IVC is usually expressed as an index to the body surface area in mm/m$^2$ [14]. Similarly, in PD populations, the IVC diameter, especially maximal diameter in quiet expiration ($IVC_e$), significantly correlates with cardiothoracic ratio and plasma ANP concentration [15]. Toprak et al. [16] proved that IVC index is a useful tool for assessing the volume status in PD patients and an independent predictor of left ventricular geometric stratification.

However, some caveats should be kept in mind: (i) there is a wide variation of IVC diameters in healthy individuals, and single measurements are not helpful; (ii) there is a significant, inverse correlation between IVC diameters and heart rate, and the precision of intravascular volume assessment is improved by correcting for the heart rate; and (iii) the presence of tricuspid insufficiency leads to unreliable results [17]. Based on these remarks, IVC diameters should be performed by an experienced cardiologist. Finally, we should keep in mind that IVC estimates only intravascular volume.

### 2.2. Biomarkers

BNP is a peptide hormone that is released primarily by the ventricular myocytes in response to myocyte stretch such as increased cardiac filling pressure. It is synthesized as an inactive prohormone (108 amino acid pro-BNP) and is cleaved into the biologically active fragment (32 amino acid c-BNP) and the N-terminal pro-B-type natriuretic peptide (76 amino acid NT-pro-BNP), and both are measurable in plasma or serum. Both provide strong prognostic information in patients with heart failure, coronary artery disease, and acute coronary syndrome. In chronic kidney disease, their concentrations are often increased due to extracellular volume expansion, concomitant heart disease, and reduced renal clearance [18]. These molecules have been associated with left ventricular hypertrophy [19, 20] and increased cardiovascular and overall mortality in HD and PD populations [21].

In ADEMEX study, only NT-proBNP levels, but not the other peptides, were alone predictive of overall survival and cardiovascular mortality of PD patients, independent of volume overload [22]. Plasma BNP levels are known to decrease significantly after a HD session, implying that volume overload is an important stimulus for BNP secretion. In PD populations, plasma BNP and NT pro-BNP levels are elevated and correlate with volume overload [23]. However, there is uncertainty if elevated levels represent more a cardiac dysfunction than volume overload [24] and doubt its use in determining volume status.

Cardiac troponins T and I (cTnT and cTnI) are subunits of the cardiac actin–myosin complex, which pass through the circulation during myocardial damage, and their detection has been used as a sensitive and specific marker of myocardial cell necrosis. Elevated serum levels of cTnT have been associated with mortality in hemodialysis [25] and CAPD patients [26]. However, as its levels are strongly associated with increased left ventricular mass [26, 27], its prognostic value is controversial. Finally, a study with HD patients from Korea compared three biomarkers (NT-proBNP, hsCRP, and cTnT) regarding the prognosis of mortality. The study concluded that NT-proBNP is a more significant prognostic factor for cardiovascular mortality than cTnT and hsCRP, whereas hsCRP is a more significant predictor than NT-proBNP and cTnT for all-cause mortality [28] So far, the data suggest that the above peptides are elevated in PD patients and correlate well with echocardiographic left ventricular parameters. Their elevated levels independently identify a subset of patients at greater risk for death, but they cannot assess volume status [29].

### 2.3. Bioelectrical impedance techniques

Bioimpedance techniques pass a low-strength alternating current into the body, and biological tissues react to the flow according to the current frequency and the properties of the tissue (this is called impedance). The two basic properties of impedance are resistance and capacitance; the former measures the flow of the electrons through the tissue, and the latter refers to how much energy is stored and released in each current alternating cycle. Resistance is proportional to the amount of fluid, while capacitance is proportional to the cell mass. Low-frequency currents (<5 kHz) pass through the ECV (they cannot pass the cell membrane), while high-frequency currents pass through both ECV and ICV compartments. There are different methods of capturing these information and illustrate them in a simple way: segmental or whole body bioimpedance spectroscopy (BIS), single or multifrequency, absolute volumes or vectors [30].

In hemodialysis populations, multifrequency bioimpedance spectroscopy (BIS) methods have been used, either segmental (measures the change of the resistance in the arm, trunk, or calf) or whole body. The segmental BIS cannot be used in PD populations, as the method presumes rapid volume reduction (as in a HD session) in order to monitor the resistance. Whole body BIS has been used widely in both populations for years in devices such as Body Composition Monitor (BCM, Fresenius Medical), Hydra (Hitron), Cyprus version 1.0 (BIA-101; RJL/Akern

Systems), and so on. The devices offer the ability to perform frequent, rapid, noninvasive assessment of the volume status.

The BCM device measures not only 50 frequencies over a range from 3 to 1000 kHz to determine the electrical resistances of TBW and the extracellular water (ECW) status, but it can also evaluate lean body weight and fat mass. This is of great interest, as there is convincing evidence for an association between volume status, inflammation, and nutritional status [31]. The ratio ECW/TBW is most widely accepted to be an index of hydration. Using population data, it also provides an estimate of the amount of overhydration (OH, measured in liters). The vector plot enables visualization of the trend toward the body composition changes, but it is inconvenient as most clinicians prefer the volume to be expressed in liters or kilos [32]. All of the bioimpedance techniques are highly reproducible and validated with dilution methods [33]. However, differences in results may occur mainly due to different devices, mathematical models used for the equations, and lack of standardization.

Numerous studies have proven the ability of BIS to estimate volume status in hemodialysis patients. In a study in HD patients [34], four different techniques for assessment of volume status were compared in order to detect the limits of each method: the measurement of vena cava diameter, vena cava collapsibility index, the blood volume drop during an ultrafiltration bolus, and the ECV determined with whole body BIS. BIS proved to have the best low-detection limit of volume overload. In PD populations, the majority of BIS-associated studies are observational ones. The largest observational longitudinal trial was performed in multiple European centers and included almost 1100 patients (IPOD-PD study) [35]. The study revealed that the majority (56.4%) of patients was overhydrated with a mean absolute value of OH 1.9 ± 2.4 l even at the start of the therapy, despite the fact the clinicians had clinically judged that 40% were normohydrated. Overhydration was commoner in males, diabetics, and fast transporters.

There is an issue if the full abdomen affects BIS measurements. Davenport et al. [36] showed that multifrequency BIS provides different measurements when the abdomen is empty. Electrical resistance increased with fluid instilled, and the BIS software algorithms overestimated muscle mass more than fat mass. This difference is greater in younger patients, in those with a poorer nutrition status (lower body mass index) and in those with a smaller fluid overload. These findings were confirmed by Arroyo et al. [37]. So, the ideal BIS measurements should be performed with empty abdomen. However, as this is clinically impractical, most authors agree that the differences in measurements are probably not clinically significant, provided they are made in a standardized way and are performed serially to document changes rather than absolute values.

In hemodialysis populations, BIS has been widely used as a tool for intervening in the evaluation of ideal dry weight [38, 39]. Similar studies in PD populations have proved the value of BCM measurements in aiding the physicians in clinical decisions [40, 41]. In a randomized controlled study in 160 continuous ambulatory peritoneal patients, fluid status was evaluated by means of repeated BIS analysis versus only clinical assessment, and the intervention group proved to be better controlled [41]. Another large randomized blinded study conducted in the United Kingdom and Shanghai [42] attempted to determine whether assessment of volume status supported by the longitudinal plot of the BI vector resulted in more stable fluid status than control subjects (where routine clinical judgment was used). Vector plot added little additional value to clinical fluid management.

There is one randomized controlled trial in HD patients, which aimed to prove that volume control guided by objective assessment of fluid overload via BIS led to improved cardiovascular outcome, namely a significant decrease in left ventricular mass index and improved blood pressure control [43]. Such a study has not yet been published in PD populations.

Several studies associated overhydration measured by BIS with mortality [44]. A retrospective study correlated hydration parameters with mortality in a PD population of above 500 patients from the United Kingdom [45]. The study used OH (l), OH/ECW ratio, and ECW/TBW ratio as volume status measurements. The first two parameters were independent predictors of mortality. In a trial from China [46], overhydration (expressed as the ratio of extracellular to intracellular water) was a predictor of mortality. The same conclusion was proved in a Korean population (overhydration was expressed as the ratio of extracellular fluid to total body fluid) [5].

BIS methods have some limitations in PD populations [47]. First, the ratio ECW/TBW is disproportionally increased due to absolute reduction in tissue mass, mainly muscle mass and abnormal tissue hydration [48, 49]. Hypoalbuminemia is another feature of PD patients, more intense than in hemodialysis patients and highly associated with comorbidity. PD patients have large protein losses through the membrane, especially high transporters and inflamed patients [49]. It is proved that in HD population without comorbidity, BIS can identify an increase in TBW and lean body mass, whereas with increasing comorbidity burden, BIS fails to demonstrate increases in tissue hydration identified only by gold standard deuterium methods [50]. As a result, in all dialysis patients, deteriorating fluid status by BIS is strongly correlated with hypoalbuminemia; this association is stronger in PD population. Secondly, clinicians should keep in mind that those absolute values of BIS measurements are based on equations derived from healthy populations (whose body composition and fluid distribution are quite different from dialysis patients). Finally, BIS cannot discriminate intravascular versus extravascular volume.

### 2.4. Lung ultrasound

It is a novel, reproducible validated technique that has been applied to estimate lung water in ESRD patients. The technique is based on the fact that when lung congestion is present, the ultrasound beam is reflected by thickened interlobular septa, generating hyperechoic artifacts between edematous septa and the overlying pleura (the so-called lung comets, considered as a ultrasound equivalent of B-lines detected in chest X-rays) (**Figure 1**). The number of these lung comets is associated with left ventricular filling pressure. Extravascular lung water is related to the ventricular filling pressure of the left ventricle [51, 52]. The technique can be easily learnt by a noncardiologist and can be performed by the bed.

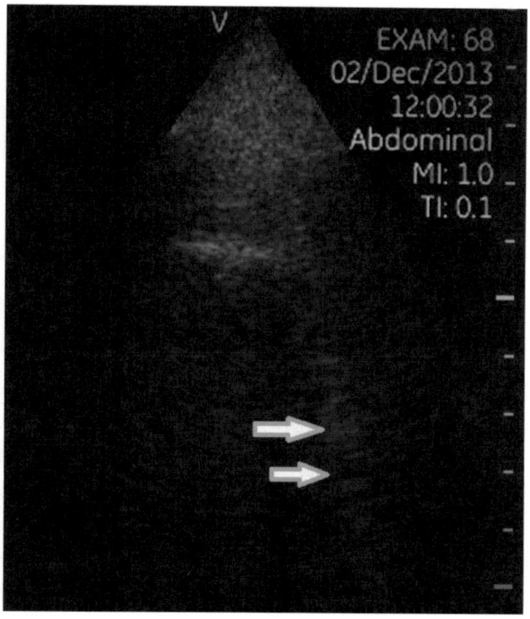


**Figure 1.** Lung ultrasound. The *arrow* shows a B-line (lung comet).

The power of the method lies in its capacity in detecting clinically asymptomatic pulmonary congestion, which is the most early and important determinator of volume overload [53]. Indeed, in a study which included HD patients [54], lung ultrasound revealed moderate-to-severe lung congestion in 63% of patients before the dialysis, even in asymptomatic ones. The number of the lung comets decreased at the end of HD session. Lung water excess was mainly associated with New York Heart Association (NYHA) functional class, left ventricular ejection fraction, left atrial volume, and pulmonary pressure. Zoccali et al. [55] proved in a multicenter study including hemodialysis patients that lung ultrasound can detect asymptomatic pulmonary congestion, and that the number of lung comets can be a strong, independent predictor of mortality and cardiac events in this population.

Another study from Romania [56] evaluated three different methods—lung ultrasonography (predialysis and postdialysis), bioimpedance spectroscopy (predialysis and postdialysis), and echocardiography (predialysis)—in order to test their prognostic value in mortality. Only predialysis lung comets score and left ventricular mass index were significant factors for survival.

However, similar studies in PD populations are sparse. Only two observational trials have been published. A multicenter study from Italy included 88 PD patients [57] and compared lung echo score, echocardiographic parameters, BIS parameters, and clinical estimation such as edema and NYHA class. Moderate-to-severe lung congestion was evident in 46% of patients, and it was mainly associated with ejection fraction and NYHA class. Edema or BIS measurements did not correlate with the number of lung score. Another study from the United Kingdom [58] assessed fluid status in 27 peritoneal dialysis patients using BIS, lung ultrasound, and N-terminal pro-brain natriuretic peptide (NT-proBNP). Contrary to the Italian study discussed above [57], the number of patients with lung congestion was lesser (7%). There was a statistically significant correlation between the lung score and NT-proBNP values, but such a correlation was not evident between lung comets and BIS. The authors conclude that as lung echocardiography and biomarkers detect intravascular and pulmonary volume excess while BIS methods estimate overall hydration status, the methods can be complementary.

## 3. Conclusions

Estimation of ideal volume status of dialysis patients is a critical purpose of everyday clinical practice, since volume overload is highly associated with mortality. The estimation of volume status should be based on objective, practical, reproducible, and by the bed methods such as bioimpedance, inferior vena cava diameter measurements, biochemical markers, and lung ultrasound. Although all these methods can estimate overhydration and do predict mortality, none so far has proved its value as an intervening tool for modifying cardiac parameters, cardiovascular events, and survival in PD patients. As these techniques estimate different fluid compartments of the body, the *information provided by the combination of them* could be complimentary and more effective in the assessment of volume status.

## Author details

Olga Balafa

Address all correspondence to: olgabalafa@gmail.com

Department of Nephrology, University Hospital of Ioannina, Ioannina, Greece

## References

[1] Agarwal R, Bouldin JM, Light RP, Garg A. Probing dry-weight improves left ventricular mass index. Am J Nephrol. 2011;33(4):373–80. Epub 2011/03/31.

[2] Kalantar-Zadeh K, Regidor DL, Kovesdy CP, Van Wyck D, Bunnapradist S, Horwich TB, et al. Fluid retention is associated with cardiovascular mortality in patients undergoing long-term hemodialysis. Circulation. 2009;119(5):671–9. Epub 2009/01/28.

[3] Parker TF, 3rd, Hakim R, Nissenson AR, Krishnan M, Bond TC, Chan K, et al. A quality initiative. Reducing rates of hospitalizations by objectively monitoring volume removal. Nephrol News Issues. 2013;27(3):30–2, 4–6. Epub 2013/04/16.

[4] Konings CJ, Kooman JP, Schonck M, Dammers R, Cheriex E, Palmans Meulemans AP, et al. Fluid status, blood pressure, and cardiovascular abnormalities in patients on peritoneal dialysis. Perit Dial Int. 2002;22(4):477–87. Epub 2002/09/27.

[5] Kang SH, Choi EW, Park JW, Cho KH, Do JY. Clinical significance of the edema index in incident peritoneal dialysis patients. PLoS One. 2016;11(1):e0147070. Epub 2016/01/20.

[6] Agarwal R, Weir MR. Dry-weight: a concept revisited in an effort to avoid medication-directed approaches for blood pressure control in hemodialysis patients. Clin J Am Soc Nephrol. 2010;5(7):1255–60. Epub 2010/05/29.

[7] Krediet RT, Smit W, Coester AM, Struijk DG. Dry body weight and ultrafiltration targets in peritoneal dialysis. Contrib Nephrol. 2009;163:90–5. Epub 2009/06/06.

[8] Agarwal R, Andersen MJ, Pratt JH. On the importance of pedal edema in hemodialysis patients. Clin J Am Soc Nephrol. 2008;3(1):153–8. Epub 2007/12/07.

[9] Wang AY, Brimble KS, Brunier G, Holt SG, Jha V, Johnson DW, et al. ISPD cardiovascular and metabolic guidelines in adult peritoneal dialysis patients part i - assessment and management of various cardiovascular risk factors. Perit Dial Int. 2015;35(4):379–87. Epub 2015/08/01.

[10] Plum J, Schoenicke G, Kleophas W, Kulas W, Steffens F, Azem A, et al. Comparison of body fluid distribution between chronic haemodialysis and peritoneal dialysis patients as assessed by biophysical and biochemical methods. Nephrol Dial Transplant. 2001;16(12):2378–85. Epub 2001/12/06.

[11] Devolder I, Verleysen A, Vijt D, Vanholder R, Van Biesen W. Body composition, hydration, and related parameters in hemodialysis versus peritoneal dialysis patients. Perit Dial Int. 2010;30(2):208–14. Epub 2010/01/19.

[12] Woodrow G, Oldroyd B, Turney JH, Davies PS, Day JM, Smith MA. Four-component model of body composition in chronic renal failure comprising dual-energy X-ray absorptiometry and measurement of total body water by deuterium oxide dilution. Clin Sci (Lond). 1996;91(6):763–9. Epub 1996/12/01.

[13] Woodrow G, Oldroyd B, Turney JH, Tompkins L, Brownjohn AM, Smith MA. Whole body and regional body composition in patients with chronic renal failure. Nephrol Dial Transplant. 1996;11(8):1613–8. Epub 1996/08/01.

[14] Cheriex EC, Leunissen KM, Janssen JH, Mooy JM, van Hooff JP. Echography of the inferior vena cava is a simple and reliable tool for estimation of 'dry weight' in haemodialysis patients. Nephrol Dial Transplant. 1989;4(6):563–8. Epub 1989/01/01.

[15] Sakurai T, Ando Y, Masunaga Y, Kusano E, Asano Y. Diameter of the inferior vena cava as an index of dry weight in patients undergoing CAPD. Perit Dial Int. 1996;16(2):183–5. Epub 1996/03/01.

[16] Toprak A, Koc M, Tezcan H, Ozener IC, Akoglu E, Oktay A. Inferior vena cava diameter determines left ventricular geometry in continuous ambulatory peritoneal dialysis patients: an echocardiographic study. Nephrol Dial Transplant. 2003;18(10):2128–33. Epub 2003/09/19.

[17] Mandelbaum A, Ritz E. Vena cava diameter measurement for estimation of dry weight in haemodialysis patients. Nephrol Dial Transplant. 1996;11 Suppl 2:24–7. Epub 1996/01/01.

[18] Crepaldi C, Lamas EI, Martino FK, Rodighiero MP, Scalzotto E, Wojewodzka-Zelezniakowicz M, et al. Bioimpedance and brain natriuretic peptide in peritoneal dialysis patients. Contrib Nephrol. 2012;178:174–81. Epub 2012/06/02.

[19] Zoccali C, Mallamaci F, Benedetto FA, Tripepi G, Parlongo S, Cataliotti A, et al. Cardiac natriuretic peptides are related to left ventricular mass and function and predict mortality in dialysis patients. J Am Soc Nephrol. 2001;12(7):1508–15. Epub 2001/06/26.

[20] Lee JA, Kim DH, Yoo SJ, Oh DJ, Yu SH, Kang ET. Association between serum n-terminal pro-brain natriuretic peptide concentration and left ventricular dysfunction and extracellular water in continuous ambulatory peritoneal dialysis patients. Perit Dial Int. 2006;26(3):360–5. Epub 2006/05/26.

[21] Wang AY, Lam CW, Yu CM, Wang M, Chan IH, Zhang Y, et al. N-terminal pro-brain natriuretic peptide: an independent risk predictor of cardiovascular congestion, mortality, and adverse cardiovascular outcomes in chronic peritoneal dialysis patients. J Am Soc Nephrol. 2007;18(1):321–30. Epub 2006/12/15.

[22] Paniagua R, Ventura MD, Avila-Diaz M, Hinojosa-Heredia H, Mendez-Duran A, Cueto-Manzano A, et al. NT-proBNP, fluid volume overload and dialysis modality are independent predictors of mortality in ESRD patients. Nephrol Dial Transplant. 2010;25(2):551–7. Epub 2009/08/15.

[23] Davenport A. Changes in N-terminal pro-brain natriuretic peptide correlate with fluid volume changes assessed by bioimpedance in peritoneal dialysis patients. Am J Nephrol. 2012;36(4):371–6. Epub 2012/10/12.

[24] Papakrivopoulou E, Booth J, Pinney J, Davenport A. Comparison of volume status in asymptomatic haemodialysis and peritoneal dialysis outpatients. Nephron Extra. 2012;2(1):48–54. Epub 2012/05/24.

[25] deFilippi C, Wasserman S, Rosanio S, Tiblier E, Sperger H, Tocchi M, et al. Cardiac troponin T and C-reactive protein for predicting prognosis, coronary atherosclerosis, and cardiomyopathy in patients undergoing long-term hemodialysis. JAMA. 2003;290(3):353–9. Epub 2003/07/17.

[26] Duman D, Tokay S, Toprak A, Duman D, Oktay A, Ozener IC, et al. Elevated cardiac troponin T is associated with increased left ventricular mass index and predicts

mortality in continuous ambulatory peritoneal dialysis patients. Nephrol Dial Transplant. 2005;20(5):962–7. Epub 2005/03/03.

[27] Mallamaci F, Zoccali C, Parlongo S, Tripepi G, Benedetto FA, Cutrupi S, et al. Diagnostic value of troponin T for alterations in left ventricular mass and function in dialysis patients. Kidney Int. 2002;62(5):1884–90. Epub 2002/10/10.

[28] Oh HJ, Lee MJ, Lee HS, Park JT, Han SH, Yoo TH, et al. NT-proBNP: is it a more significant risk factor for mortality than troponin T in incident hemodialysis patients? Medicine (Baltimore). 2014;93(27):e241. Epub 2014/12/17.

[29] Garg R, Singh A, Khaja A, Martin A, Aggarwal K. How does volume status affect BNP and troponin levels as markers of cardiovascular status in peritoneal dialysis? Congest Heart Fail. 2009;15(5):240–4. Epub 2009/09/16.

[30] Davies SJ, Davenport A. The role of bioimpedance and biomarkers in helping to aid clinical decision-making of volume assessments in dialysis patients. Kidney Int. 2014;86(3):489–96. Epub 2014/06/12.

[31] Cheng LT, Tang W, Wang T. Strong association between volume status and nutritional status in peritoneal dialysis patients. Am J Kidney Dis. 2005;45(5):891–902. Epub 2005/04/30.

[32] Piccoli A. Whole body--single frequency bioimpedance. Contrib Nephrol. 2005;149:150–61. Epub 2005/05/07.

[33] Konings CJ, Kooman JP, Schonck M, Cox-Reijven PL, van Kreel B, Gladziwa U, et al. Assessment of fluid status in peritoneal dialysis patients. Perit Dial Int. 2002;22(6):683–92. Epub 2003/01/31.

[34] Kraemer M, Rode C, Wizemann V. Detection limit of methods to assess fluid status changes in dialysis patients. Kidney Int. 2006;69(9):1609–20. Epub 2006/02/28.

[35] Ronco C, Verger C, Crepaldi C, Pham J, De Los Rios T, Gauly A, et al. Baseline hydration status in incident peritoneal dialysis patients: the initiative of patient outcomes in dialysis (IPOD-PD study)dagger. Nephrol Dial Transplant. 2015;30(5):849–58. Epub 2015/03/13.

[36] Davenport A. Effect of intra-abdominal dialysate on bioimpedance-derived fluid volume status and body composition measurements in peritoneal dialysis patients. Perit Dial Int. 2013;33(5):578–9. Epub 2013/10/18.

[37] Arroyo D, Panizo N, Abad S, Vega A, Rincon A, de Jose AP, et al. Intraperitoneal fluid overestimates hydration status assessment by bioimpedance spectroscopy. Perit Dial Int. 2015;35(1):85–9. Epub 2014/03/04.

[38] Liu L, Zhu F, J GR, Thijssen S, Sipahioglu MH, Wystrychowski G, et al. Determination of fluid status in haemodialysis patients with whole body and calf bioimpedance techniques. Nephrology (Carlton). 2012;17(2):131–40. Epub 2011/09/29.

[39] Passauer J, Petrov H, Schleser A, Leicht J, Pucalka K. Evaluation of clinical dry weight assessment in haemodialysis patients using bioimpedance spectroscopy: a cross-sectional study. Nephrol Dial Transplant. 2010;25(2):545–51. Epub 2009/10/08.

[40] van Biesen W, Claes K, Covic A, Fan S, Lichodziejewska-Niemierko M, Schoder V, et al. A multicentric, international matched pair analysis of body composition in peritoneal dialysis versus haemodialysis patients. Nephrol Dial Transplant. 2013;28(10): 2620–8. Epub 2013/10/01.

[41] Luo YJ, Lu XH, Woods F, Wang T. Volume control in peritoneal dialysis patients guided by bioimpedance spectroscopy assessment. Blood Purif. 2011;31(4):296–302. Epub 2011/01/19.

[42] T an BK, Yu Z, Fang W, Lin A, Ni Z, Qian J, et al. Longitudinal bioimpedance vector plots add little value to fluid management of peritoneal dialysis patients. Kidney Int. 2016;89(2):487-497. Epub 2016/01/22

[43] Hur E, Usta M, Toz H, Asci G, Wabel P, Kahvecioglu S, et al. Effect of fluid management guided by bioimpedance spectroscopy on cardiovascular parameters in hemodialysis patients: a randomized controlled trial. Am J Kidney Dis. 2013;61(6):957–65. Epub 2013/02/19.

[44] Koh KH, Wong HS, Go KW, Morad Z. Normalized bioimpedance indices are better predictors of outcome in peritoneal dialysis patients. Perit Dial Int. 2011;31(5):574–82. Epub 2010/07/02.

[45] O'Lone EL, Visser A, Finney H, Fan SL. Clinical significance of multi-frequency bioimpedance spectroscopy in peritoneal dialysis patients: independent predictor of patient survival. Nephrol Dial Transplant. 2014;29(7):1430–7. Epub 2014/03/07.

[46] Chen W, Guo LJ, Wang T. Extracellular water/intracellular water is a strong predictor of patient survival in incident peritoneal dialysis patients. Blood Purif. 2007;25(3):260–6. Epub 2007/04/13.

[47] Tan BK, Chan C, Davies SJ. Achieving euvolemia in peritoneal dialysis patients: a surprisingly difficult proposition. Semin Dial. 2010;23(5):456–61. Epub 2010/11/03.

[48] Woodrow G, Devine Y, Cullen M, Lindley E. Application of bioelectrical impedance to clinical assessment of body composition in peritoneal dialysis. Perit Dial Int. 2007;27(5): 496–502. Epub 2007/08/21.

[49] John B, Tan BK, Dainty S, Spanel P, Smith D, Davies SJ. Plasma volume, albumin, and fluid status in peritoneal dialysis patients. Clin J Am Soc Nephrol. 2010;5(8):1463–70. Epub 2010/06/12.

[50] Chan C, McIntyre C, Smith D, Spanel P, Davies SJ. Combining near-subject absolute and relative measures of longitudinal hydration in hemodialysis. Clin J Am Soc Nephrol. 2009;4(11):1791–8. Epub 2009/10/08.

[51] Picano E, Frassi F, Agricola E, Gligorova S, Gargani L, Mottola G. Ultrasound lung comets: a clinically useful sign of extravascular lung water. J Am Soc Echocardiogr. 2006;19(3):356–63. Epub 2006/02/28.

[52] Gargani L, Frassi F, Soldati G, Tesorio P, Gheorghiade M, Picano E. Ultrasound lung comets for the differential diagnosis of acute cardiogenic dyspnoea: a comparison with natriuretic peptides. Eur J Heart Fail. 2008;10(1):70–7. Epub 2007/12/14.

[53] Zoccali C, Puntorieri E, Mallamaci F. Lung congestion as a hidden threat in end-stage kidney disease: a call to action. Nephrol Dial Transplant. 2013;28(11):2657–60. Epub 2013/10/31.

[54] Mallamaci F, Benedetto FA, Tripepi R, Rastelli S, Castellino P, Tripepi G, et al. Detection of pulmonary congestion by chest ultrasound in dialysis patients. JACC Cardiovasc Imaging. 2010;3(6):586–94. Epub 2010/06/15.

[55] Zoccali C, Torino C, Tripepi R, Tripepi G, D'Arrigo G, Postorino M, et al. Pulmonary congestion predicts cardiac events and mortality in ESRD. J Am Soc Nephrol. 2013;24(4):639–46. Epub 2013/03/02.

[56] Siriopol D, Voroneanu L, Hogas S, Apetrii M, Gramaticu A, Dumea R, et al. Bioimpedance analysis versus lung ultrasonography for optimal risk prediction in hemodialysis patients. Int J Cardiovasc Imaging. 2016;32(2):263–70. Epub 2015/10/03.

[57] Panuccio V, Enia G, Tripepi R, Torino C, Garozzo M, Battaglia GG, et al. Chest ultrasound and hidden lung congestion in peritoneal dialysis patients. Nephrol Dial Transplant. 2012;27(9):3601–5. Epub 2012/05/11.

[58] Paudel K, Kausik T, Visser A, Ramballi C, Fan SL. Comparing lung ultrasound with bioimpedance spectroscopy for evaluating hydration in peritoneal dialysis patients. Nephrology (Carlton). 2015;20(1):1–5. Epub 2014/09/19.

# Chapter 6

# Diagnosis and Management of Exit Site Infection in Peritoneal Dialysis Patients

Desmond Y.H. Yap and Terence Yip

Additional information is available at the end of the chapter

http://dx.doi.org/10.5772/63769

**Abstract**

Exit site infection (ESI) is an important clinical problem in peritoneal dialysis (PD) patients and is a significant cause of peritonitis and catheter loss. While most ESIs are caused by skin commensals, rising incidence of atypical and resilient organisms such as mycobacteria, *Pseudomonas* and *Burkholderia* species has been observed. The diagnosis and management of these emerging pathogen remain difficult and poorly defined. This chapter highlights the evaluation and management of ESI in PD patients. The clinical features, microbiology, and ultrasonographic findings are discussed. The general and specific management of ESI due to different organisms will also be elaborated. ESI is usually a clinical diagnosis, but the use of bedside ultrasound can help assess for any collection around the cuff and tunnel tract involvement. Topical prophylaxis remains an effective way to prevent ESI. While the majority ESIs are related to skin flora and can be managed successfully by topical or systemic antimicrobials, clinicians should be alert to the emergence of resistant and atypical microorganisms. Surgical treatment should be reserved for ESI refractory to medical treatment or those with associated peritonitis.

**Keywords:** exit site infection, peritoneal dialysis, diagnosis, prophylaxis, management

## 1. Introduction

Peritoneal dialysis (PD) is an important modality of renal replacement therapy and is gaining popularity in both developed and developing countries [1]. While PD is associated with lower treatment costs and better patient autonomy when compared to hemodialysis, the practice of PD is also burdened with various infectious and noninfectious complications. PD catheter (also known as Tenckhoff catheter) is an essential device for the performance of PD exchanges. However, the implantation of a PD catheter is associated with infective complications such as exit site infection (ESI), tunnel tract infections, and peritonitis. Repeated or fulminant PD peritonitis heralds adverse clinical outcomes such as catheter loss, peritoneal failure and patient mortality [2–4]. Therefore, prevention of peritonitis plays a crucial role in the care of PD patients. In this context, ESI constitutes a significant risk factor for peritonitis, and thus prevention and appropriate management of ESI can substantially diminish the risk of PD-related peritonitis [2–5], and thus improve overall patient outcomes.

## 2. Pathogenesis and microbiology of exit site infection in peritoneal dialysis patients

In most PD patients, colonization with microorganisms occurs shortly after the implantation of PD catheter. Colonization does not equate clinical infection, but predisposes PD patients to ESI, especially after exit site traumatization. Bacterial colonization of exit site is frequently followed by formation of biofilm, which promote further bacterial growth and void the colonizing microorganisms from antimicrobial treatments. The organisms that colonize the exit site are often the same pathogens responsible for ESI [6]. Common pathogens to cause ESI in PD patients include *Staphylococcus aureus, coagulase negative staphylococcus (CNS), Pseudomonas aeruginosa,* and other Gram-negative bacilli [2]. With the widespread application of exit site prophylaxis, there is a shift in causative agents for ESI. For instance, some studies have suggested that the use of mupirocin or gentamicin ointment may predispose patients to fungal exit site infections [7, 8]. There is also emergence of exotic organisms such as atypical mycobacteria, *corynebacteria* as well as *Burkholderia* species to cause ESI [2, 9–11]. Furthermore, the development of antibiotics resistance remains an important concern in the management of ESI.

### 2.1. Staphylococcus aureus

*S. aureus* is a Gram-positive coccus and a common skin commensal. It is one of the commonest causative agents for ESI in PD patients, and accounts for over 50% of ESI cases [6]. In general, *S. aureus* can be categorized into *methicillin-sensitive S. aureus (MSSA)* and *methicillin-resistant S. aureus (MRSA). Methicillin-resistant S. aureus (MRSA)* refer to strains of *S. aureus* that have developed resistance to β-lactam antibiotics including penicillinase-resistant penicillins (methicillin, cloxacillin, etc.) and cephalosporins. One national survey conducted among nephrology units in the United States has reported that over 40% of isolates of *S. aureus* belong to the *MRSA* strains [12]. Diabetes mellitus, increased age, immunocompromised state and protracted hospital stay are common and important risk factors for *MRSA* infections [13]. *MRSA* is a frequent cause of ESI, tunnel tract infection and peritonitis in PD patients, and is associated with appreciable morbidity and mortality in dialysis populations [14–16].

### 2.2. Coagulase-negative staphylococcus

*Coagulase-negative staphylococci (CNS)* are skin flora that can cause ESI. *Staphylococcus epidermidis* and *Staphylococcus saprophyticus* are common *CNS*, and the former accounts for roughly 20% of all ESI [6]. Other CNS that can cause ESI include *Staphylococcus lugdunensis* and

*Staphylococcus warneri* [17]. While most *CNS* will respond to first-generation cephalosporins or penicillinase-resistant penicillin, there is growing prevalence for *methicillin-resistant CNS (MRCNS)*.

### 2.3. Other Gram-positive organisms

*Corynebacterium* species (e.g., *diphtheroids*) are common skin commensals which exhibit intrinsic resistance to many commonly used antibiotics such as β-lactams, clindamycin, macrolides, quinolones and gentamicin [18]. Other Gram-positive bacteria that can be associated with ESI include *streptococcal* species (e.g., *Streptococcus sanguinus*) and *enterococcal* species [2, 17].

### 2.4. Pseudomonas aeruginosa

*P. aeruginosa* is a Gram-negative rod-shaped bacterium that commonly causes ESI in PD patients and is responsible for 8% of all ESI [6]. *P. aeruginosa* is a notorious for its ubiquity and intrinsic resistance to many commonly used antibiotics. Furthermore, *P. aeruginosa* is also well recognized for biofilm formation which contributes the persistence of infection. With these properties, *P. aeruginosa* often causes refractory ESI, requires prolonged antibiotics and is also associated with high risk of catheter loss [19, 20]. Moreover, around 20% of patients develop *P. aeruginosa* peritonitis several months after the resolution of ESI [19].

### 2.5. Other Gram-negative organisms and anaerobes

Gram-negative bacilli are also important causes of ESI, and *Escherichia coli* accounts for about 4% of all cases of ESI [6]. Other Gram-negative organisms that can cause ESI include *Klebsiella pneumoniae, Enterobacter* species and *Proteus mirabilis* [17]. The emergence of extended spectrum β-lactamase (ESBL)-producing Gram-negative bacilli is an escalating threat in the management of ESI. Other emerging pathogens to cause ESI include *Burkholderia cepacia*, which is a hardy nonfermenting Gram-negative organism [10, 11]. Its intrinsic resistance to multiple commercially available antibiotics and easy transmissibility renders it a growing problem in dialysis units. Although, *B. cepacia* is associated with low risk of tunnel tract infection or peritonitis, it is associated with a high rate of recurrence after successful antibiotics treatment [11]. Occasionally, anaerobes (e.g., *micrococcus*) can be also isolated from ESI in PD patients [17].

### 2.6. Mycobacterium

Rapidly growing atypical mycobacteria are more frequent causative agents for ESI than *Mycobacterium tuberculosis*. Atypical mycobacteria that commonly cause ESI include *M. chelonae, M. fortuitum* and *M. abscessus* [9, 21]. It is postulated that the use of gentamicin may predispose patients to atypical mycobacterial infections due to selection pressure on other microorganisms [9]. ESI due to atypical mycobacteria require prolonged systemic antimicrobial treatments and is associated with high rates of catheter loss [21]. Although dialysis patients are at risk of *M. tuberculosis* infection, ESI due to *M. tuberculosis* is not common and usually occur as part of a disseminated tuberculosis infection.

### 2.7. Fungi

Fungal ESI is a rare cause of ESI, and *Candida* species (being skin flora) are the commonest fungi isolated in this context. Some literatures have suggested that the use of mupirocin or gentamicin ointment prophylaxis might increase the risk of fungal ESI [7, 8].

## 3. Clinical features and evaluation of exit site infection in peritoneal dialysis patients

ESI is characterized by purulent discharge from the exit site, and with or without erythema or induration at the exit site [2, 22]. Although erythema around the PD catheter in the absence of purulent discharge may represent early signs of ESI, this can also be normal skin reaction to recently implanted PD catheter or exit site traumatization. The presence of crust around the exit site or positive cultures from exit site without signs of inflammation, however, does not indicate an ESI. The spectrum of severity of ESI can range from increased crust formation, to erythema around the exit site, to serous or purulent discharge, to abscess formation, and to tunnel tract involvement. In this context, different grading systems have been proposed to document the clinical severity of ESI [22, 23]. Assessment of the exit site involves gross inspection of the exit site, palpation of the tunnel tract and expression of discharge from the exit site. The discharge should be sent for microbiological examination (Gram smear, culture and sensitivity pattern), which can guide further treatment decisions. Ultrasonography has also been used to assess ESI, especially with regard to local collections and tunnel tract involvements [24]. In this context, sonolucent zone (>1 mm thick) surrounding the external cuff after a course of appropriate antimicrobial therapy and the involvement of the internal cuff portends adverse clinical outcomes [24].

## 4. Prevention of exit site infection in peritoneal dialysis patients

Proper care of the exit site constitutes an integral component in the prevention of ESI. In the early postoperative period (~first 2 weeks), the exit site should be kept dry until it is well healed [22]. The exit site should be covered with sterile dressing and the change of dressing should be performed by experienced nursing staff before the patient is properly trained. After completion of PD training, the patient should be able to clean the exit site with antiseptic agents (e.g., povidone iodine or chlorhexidine) on daily or alternate day basis, and the exit site be constantly covered with sterile dressings [22].

Hand hygiene is a key measure to decrease ESI in PD patients. Good hand hygiene practices should be undertaken by patients, helpers and healthcare providers during routine handling of the PD catheter and its exit site [25]. In this regard, 70% alcohol-based hand rub is the most effective hand-sanitizing agent to be used before and after the handing of PD catheter and its exit site [26]. Alternative hand-sanitizing agents include antimicrobial-containing (e.g., 4% chlorhexidine) soap [26].

*S. aureus* is a frequent pathogen to cause ESI, and associated with PD-related peritonitis and catheter loss [27]. The application of exit site prophylaxis can markedly diminish the PD-related *S. aureus* infection and thus should be undertaken in all PD patients [7, 28]. In this context, topical mupirocin has demonstrated its effectiveness as prophylaxis for *S. aureus* ESI [7, 28–32]. In one previous observational study involving more than 700 new PD patients, the use of topical mupirocin as exit site prophylaxis leads to a significant reduction in both ESI (0.168 vs. 0.156 episodes per patient-year) and peritonitis (0.443 vs. 0.339 episodes per patient-year) [32]. Subsequent meta-analyses corroborated these observations and highlighted that topical mupirocin was associated with 60–70% decrease in both *S. aureus* ESI and peritonitis [29, 33]. The administration of intranasal mupirocin has been investigated in a large multi-center trial, which showed that intranasal mupirocin in PD patients with confirmed nasal *S. aureus* carriage prevent ESI but not peritonitis [34]. However, data that compared intranasal versus exit-site route of mupirocin prophylaxis are lacking.

Although the exit site prophylaxis with mupirocin has curbed *S. aureus* infection in PD patients, *P. aeruginosa* remains an important culprit for ESI. Gentamicin is an aminoglycoside that demonstrates good activity against both *S. aureus* and *P. aeruginosa*. The application of daily gentamicin ointment versus daily mupirocin ointment as exit site prophylaxis has been investigated in a multi-center double-blind randomized clinical trial. The results demonstrated that gentamicin and mupirocin are similarly effective in preventing *S. aureus* ESI but the former conferred an advantage on preventing *Pseudomonas* ESI. Notwithstanding, liberal administration of gentamicin ointment as exit site prophylaxis might predispose PD patients to fungal ESI. Other novel prophylactic therapies for PD exit site include MediHoney and Polysporin triple (bacitracin, gramicidin and polymixin B) ointment [8, 35].

## 5. Management of exit site infection in peritoneal dialysis patients

### 5.1. General principles (Figure 1)

Exit site care and local dressing constitutes the cornerstone in the management of ESI. Topical antiseptics (e.g., mupirocin, gentamicin ointment) are all viable options for dressing of exit sites. Other alternatives such as hypertonic saline solution can be considered in selected cases (e.g., *P. aeruginosa* ESI). Empirical oral or intravenous antibiotics should be initiated after appropriate microbiological samples have been obtained and should always cover *S. aureus*. However, the choice of empirical antimicrobial treatment should also take into consideration the likely organism involved, medical background of the patients, previous culture and resistance profile of organisms isolated from the patient and the local antibiotics susceptibility/resistance pattern [2]. In general, first-generation cephalosporins or penicillinase-resistant penicillins can be used as initial treatment for ESI in PD patients [2]. The choice of antibiotics and duration of treatment can be further modified when the culture identity and the susceptibility/resistance profile are available. Trimming/shaving of the external cuff can be considered if the external cuff is partially or fully protruding outside the exit site [6, 36] (**Figure 2**). Catheters should be removed when there is recurrent infection due to the same organism, ESI refractory to medical therapy, presence of tunnel tract abscess or associated peritonitis [2]. Most patients will require temporary hemodialysis while pending catheter reinsertion, simultaneous removal and reimplantation of PD catheter can be considered in selected cases to avoid bridging hemodialysis [37]. However, such approach is not advisable when there is also concomitant active peritonitis.

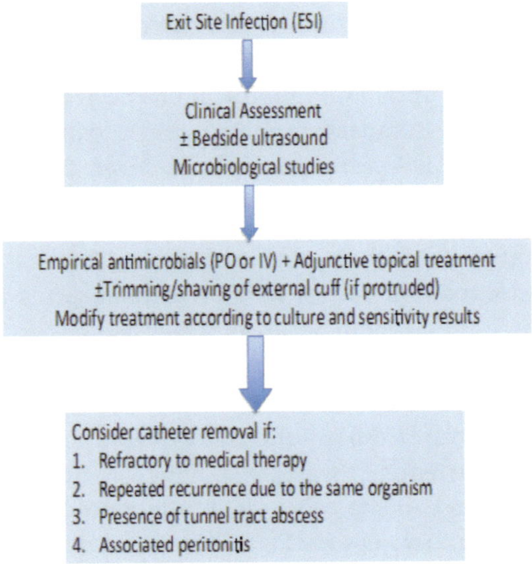


**Figure 1.** Management algorithm for exit site infection in peritoneal dialysis patients.

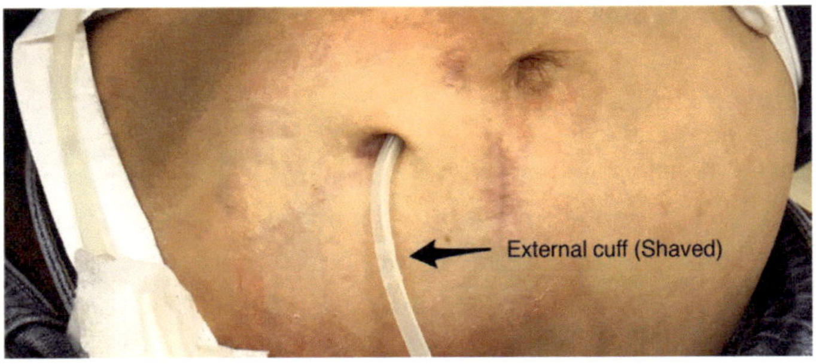


**Figure 2.** PD catheter after shaving of external catheter.

## 5.2. Management of exit site infection due to specific organisms

### *5.2.1. Methicillin-sensitive or resistant S. aureus*

First-generation cephalosporins (e.g., cephazolin) or penicillinase-resistant penicillins (e.g., cloxacillin) can be used in MSSA ESI [2]. Parenteral vancomycin has established clinical efficacy in the treatment of MRSA ESI, tunnel tract tunnel infection and peritonitis in PD patients [2]. In this context, intravenous (IV) vancomycin (1 g every 5–7 days for a minimum of 14 days) is a standard treatment of MRSA exit site or tunnel tract infection in PD patients [2]. However, rising MIC to vancomycin remains a valid concern for the use of vancomycin in MRSA infection. Other viable choices for MRSA infections in PD patients include teicoplanin, daptomycin, linezolid, tigecycline, and quinupristin-dalfopristin. Teicoplanin is a glycopeptide that exhibits activity and efficacy profile resembling vancomycin, and has the merit of longer half-life and superior tolerability than vancomycin. Daptomycin is an approved treatment of complicated MRSA soft-tissue infections and bacteremia (with or without infection endocarditis) in a dosage of 6 mg/kg/day [38, 39]. In CKD stage 4 or 5 patients, the dosage of daptomycin should remain unchanged but the frequency be reduced to every 48 hours [40]. Linezolid (600 mg B.I.D., IV or PO) can be used for the treatment of MRSA skin infection as well as community- or hospital-acquired MRSA pneumonia [41, 42]. No dosage modification is required for linezolid in dialysis patients but one should be aware of the side effects such as myelosuppression and lactic acidosis [42]. Tigecycline demonstrates promising *in vitro* activity against most *MRSA* strains and is an approved treatment for MRSA skin and intra-abdominal infections [43–45]. No dosage reduction is required for the use of tigecycline in PD patients is another added advantage. Quinupristin-dalfopristin is an approved treatment for *MRSA* soft-tissue infections with no dosage modification in renal failure patients. However, its data in PD patients are relatively scarce [40]. Clindamycin is not recommended for *MRSA* ESI in PD patients due to its unreliable activity against *MRSA* acquired nosocomially [42, 46]. Other emerging antimicrobials for MRSA infections include lipoglycopeptides dalbavancin, telavancin and oritavancin as well as newer generation cephalosporins such as ceftobiprole and ceftaroline [43, 44, 47]. The data on these novel agents for MRSA ESI, however, remain limited in PD patients.

#### *5.2.2. Pseudomonas aeruginosa*

Topical treatments (e.g., gentamicin ointment) can be used as adjunctive treatment for mild *P. aeruginosa* ESI [2]. Other alternatives include hypertonic saline although such therapy is not a standard practice [22]. Previous studies have reported the efficacy of oral fluoroquinolones (e.g., ciprofloxacin or levofloxacin) for the treatment of ESI due to *P. aeruginosa* [2, 19, 48]. Current standard-of-care therapy for the ESI consisted of oral fluoroquinolones (e.g., ciprofloxacin 500 mg B.I.D) and local application of antiseptic agents to the exit site [2, 19, 48]. Intravenous antibiotics should be used in severe ESI due to *P. aeruginosa* [2]. Choices of intravenous antibiotics include third- or fourth-generation cephalosporins (e.g., ceftazidime and cefepime), ticarcillin/clavulanate, piperacillin (with or without tazobactam) and carbapenems. The optimal duration of antibiotics treatment should be at least 2–3 weeks [2]. Catheter removal should be considered in cases with refractory ESI which respond poorly to medical treatment or associated peritonitis [2]. Up to 50–80% of patients with ESI due to *P. aeruginosa* ESI respond to medical therapy, while approximately 20–36% would require catheter removal [19, 48].

*5.2.3. Other Gram-negative organisms*

In general, ESI due to Gram-negative organisms are susceptible to second- or third-generation cephalosporins [2, 22]. However, there is increasing prevalence of ESBL-producing Gram-negative organisms. Carbapenems should be considered in patients with previous history of ESBL-producing organisms or when the ESI do not respond to second- or third-generation cephalosporins [2]. *B. cepacia* are generally susceptible to ceftazidime (95.5%), piperacillin/ tazobactam (95.5%) and pipercillin (90.9%) [11]. While most patients with *B. cepacia* ESI will respond to medical therapy, a high rate of recurrence is observed. Similar to *P. aeruginosa* ESI, the duration of treatment for *B. cepacia* ESI should be extended up to 3 weeks.

*5.2.4. Mycobacterium*

The treatment regimen for atypical mycobacterium ESI is dependent on the organisms identified as well as the susceptibility/resistance profiles. In general, the regimen should consist of at least two or more antimycobacterial agents (e.g., parenteral aminoglycosides, fluoroquinolones, tetracyclines and macrolides), and prolonged therapy is generally required [2, 21]. In this context, a combination of oral fluoroquinolones, tetracyclines (doxycycline or minocycline), macrolides (clarithromycin or azithromycin) or cotrimoxazole can be administered for *M. fortuitum* ESI [21, 49]. Clarithromycin, in combination with doxycycline or ciprofloxacin, is commonly used in localities where most *M. chelonae* are susceptible to macrolides [21]. The treatment regimen for *M. abscessus* should comprise clarithromycin plus either amikacin or high-dose cefoxitin [21]. The prolonged administration of aminoglycosides and macrolides is associated with ototoxicity and cardiac arrhythmia (QT prolongation) in PD patients. Approximately 44% of patients will respond to medical therapy and catheter removal should be considered in patients with refractory mycobacterial ESI.

*5.2.5. Fungal exit site infection*

Fungal ESI is rare clinical entity and there are limited data regarding the optimal management of fungal ESI. It is important to exclude contamination when fungus is isolated from the exit site, and removal of PD catheter should be considered if there is established fungal ESI to avoid fungal peritonitis.

## Author details

Desmond Y.H. Yap[1*] and Terence Yip[2]

*Address all correspondence to: desmondy@hku.hk

1 Nephrology Division, Department of Medicine, Queen Mary Hospital, The University of Hong Kong, Hong Kong

2 Renal Unit, Tung Wah Hospital, Hong Kong

http://dx.doi.org/10.5772/63769

## References

[1] Jain AK, Blake P, Cordy P, Garg AX. Global trends in rates of peritoneal dialysis. J Am Soc Nephrol 2012;23:533–44.

[2] Li PK, Szeto CC, Piraino B, et al. Peritoneal dialysis-related infections recommendations: 2010 update. Perit Dial Int 2010;30:393–423.

[3] Piraino B, Bernardini J, Sorkin M. The influence of peritoneal catheter exit-site infections on peritonitis, tunnel infections, and catheter loss in patients on continuous ambulatory peritoneal dialysis. Am J Kidney Dis 1986;8:436–40.

[4] Piraino B, Bernardini J, Sorkin M. Catheter infections as a factor in the transfer of continuous ambulatory peritoneal dialysis patients to hemodialysis. Am J Kidney Dis 1989;13:365–9.

[5] Gupta B, Bernardini J, Piraino B. Peritonitis associated with exit site and tunnel infections. Am J Kidney Dis 1996;28:415–9.

[6] Scalamogna A, Castelnovo C, De Vecchi A, Ponticelli C. Exit-site and tunnel infections in continuous ambulatory peritoneal dialysis patients. Am J Kidney Dis 1991;18:674–7.

[7] Bernardini J, Bender F, Florio T, et al. Randomized, double-blind trial of antibiotic exit site cream for prevention of exit site infection in peritoneal dialysis patients. J Am Soc Nephrol 2005;16:539–45.

[8] McQuillan RF, Chiu E, Nessim S, et al. A randomized controlled trial comparing mupirocin and polysporin triple ointments in peritoneal dialysis patients: the MP3 Study. Clin J Am Soc Nephrol 2012;7:297–303.

[9] Tse KC, Lui SL, Cheng VC, Yip TP, Lo WK. A cluster of rapidly growing mycobacterial peritoneal dialysis catheter exit-site infections. Am J Kidney Dis 2007;50:e1–5.

[10] Yap DY, Choy CB, Mok MM, Wong TK, Chan TM. Burkholderia cepacia-an uncommon cause of exit-site infection in a peritoneal dialysis patient. Perit Dial Int 2014;34:471–2.

[11] Yap DY, Chan JF, Yip T, et al. Burkholderia cepacia exit-site infection in peritoneal dialysis patients-clinical characteristics and treatment outcomes. Perit Dial Int 2015. [Epub ahead of print].

[12] Klevens RM, Edwards JR, Andrus ML, et al. Dialysis Surveillance Report: National Healthcare Safety Network (NHSN)-data summary for 2006. Semin Dial 2008;21:24–8.

[13] Vandecasteele SJ, Boelaert JR, De Vriese AS. *Staphylococcus aureus* infections in hemodialysis: what a nephrologist should know. Clin J Am Soc Nephrol 2009;4:1388–400.

[14] Cosgrove SE, Qi Y, Kaye KS, Harbarth S, Karchmer AW, Carmeli Y. The impact of methicillin resistance in *Staphylococcus aureus* bacteremia on patient outcomes: mortal-

ity, length of stay, and hospital charges. Infect Control Hosp Epidemiol 2005;26:166–74.

[15] Reed SD, Friedman JY, Engemann JJ, et al. Costs and outcomes among hemodialysis-dependent patients with methicillin-resistant or methicillin-susceptible *Staphylococcus aureus* bacteremia. Infect Control Hosp Epidemiol 2005;26:175–83.

[16] Shurland S, Zhan M, Bradham DD, Roghmann MC. Comparison of mortality risk associated with bacteremia due to methicillin-resistant and methicillin-susceptible *Staphylococcus aureus*. Infect Control Hosp Epidemiol 2007;28:273–9.

[17] Pihl M, Davies JR, Johansson AC, Svensater G. Bacteria on catheters in patients undergoing peritoneal dialysis. Perit Dial Int 2013;33:51–9.

[18] Soriano F, Zapardiel J, Nieto E. Antimicrobial susceptibilities of Corynebacterium species and other non-spore-forming gram-positive bacilli to 18 antimicrobial agents. Antimicrob Agents Chemother 1995;39:208–14.

[19] Kazmi HR, Raffone FD, Kliger AS, Finkelstein FO. Pseudomonas exit site infections in continuous ambulatory peritoneal dialysis patients. J Am Soc Nephrol 1992;2:1498–501.

[20] Szabo T, Siccion Z, Izatt S, Vas SI, Bargman J, Oreopoulos DG. Outcome of *Pseudomonas aeruginosa* exit-site and tunnel infections: a single center's experience. Adv Perit Dial 1999;15:209–12.

[21] Lo MW, Mak SK, Wong YY, et al. Atypical mycobacterial exit-site infection and peritonitis in peritoneal dialysis patients on prophylactic exit-site gentamicin cream. Perit Dial Int 2013;33:267–72.

[22] Piraino B, Bailie GR, Bernardini J, et al. Peritoneal dialysis-related infections recommendations: 2005 update. Perit Dial Int 2005;25:107–31.

[23] Twardowski ZJ, Prowant BF. Current approach to exit-site infections in patients on peritoneal dialysis. Nephrol Dial Transplant 1997;12:1284–95.

[24] Kwan TH, Tong MK, Siu YP, Leung KT, Luk SH, Cheung YK. Ultrasonography in the management of exit site infections in peritoneal dialysis patients. Nephrology (Carlton) 2004;9:348–52.

[25] Piraino B, Bernardini J, Brown E, et al. ISPD position statement on reducing the risks of peritoneal dialysis-related infections. Perit Dial Int 2011;31:614–30.

[26] (CDC) USDoHaHSCfDCaP. Hand hygiene in healthcare settings (http://www.cdc.gov/Handhygiene). Atlanta, GA, USA, 2011.

[27] Piraino B. A review of *Staphylococcus aureus* exit-site and tunnel infections in peritoneal dialysis patients. Am J Kidney Dis 1990;16:89–95.

[28] Thodis E, Bhaskaran S, Pasadakis P, Bargman JM, Vas SI, Oreopoulos DG. Decrease in *Staphylococcus aureus* exit-site infections and peritonitis in CAPD patients by local

application of mupirocin ointment at the catheter exit site. Perit Dial Int 1998;18:261–70.

[29] Xu G, Tu W, Xu C. Mupirocin for preventing exit-site infection and peritonitis in patients undergoing peritoneal dialysis. Nephrol Dial Transplant 2010;25:587–92.

[30] Piraino B, Bernardini J, Florio T, Fried L. *Staphylococcus aureus* prophylaxis and trends in gram-negative infections in peritoneal dialysis patients. Perit Dial Int 2003;23:456–9.

[31] Mahajan S, Tiwari SC, Kalra V, et al. Effect of local mupirocin application on exit-site infection and peritonitis in an Indian peritoneal dialysis population. Perit Dial Int 2005;25:473–7.

[32] Lim CT, Wong KS, Foo MW. The impact of topical mupirocin on peritoneal dialysis infection in Singapore General Hospital. Nephrol Dial Transplant 2005;20:2202–6.

[33] Tacconelli E, Carmeli Y, Aizer A, Ferreira G, Foreman MG, D'Agata EM. Mupirocin prophylaxis to prevent *Staphylococcus aureus* infection in patients undergoing dialysis: a meta-analysis. Clin Infect Dis 2003;37:1629–38.

[34] Nasal mupirocin prevents *Staphylococcus aureus* exit-site infection during peritoneal dialysis. Mupirocin Study Group. J Am Soc Nephrol 1996;7:2403–8.

[35] Johnson DW, Clark C, Isbel NM, et al. The honeypot study protocol: a randomized controlled trial of exit-site application of medihoney antibacterial wound gel for the prevention of catheter-associated infections in peritoneal dialysis patients. Perit Dial Int 2009;29:303–9.

[36] Scalamogna A, De Vecchi A, Maccario M, Castelnovo C, Ponticelli C. Cuff-shaving procedure. A rescue treatment for exit-site infection unresponsive to medical therapy. Nephrol Dial Transplant 1995;10:2325–7.

[37] Lui SL, Yip T, Tse KC, Lam MF, Lai KN, Lo WK. Treatment of refractory *Pseudomonas aeruginosa* exit-site infection by simultaneous removal and reinsertion of peritoneal dialysis catheter. Perit Dial Int 2005;25:560–3.

[38] Boucher HW, Sakoulas G. Perspectives on Daptomycin resistance, with emphasis on resistance in *Staphylococcus aureus*. Clin Infect Dis 2007;45:601–8.

[39] Fowler VG, Jr., Boucher HW, Corey GR, et al. Daptomycin versus standard therapy for bacteremia and endocarditis caused by *Staphylococcus aureus*. N Engl J Med 2006;355:653–65.

[40] Salzer W. Antimicrobial-resistant gram-positive bacteria in PD peritonitis and the newer antibiotics used to treat them. Perit Dial Int 2005;25:313–9.

[41] Moellering RC. Linezolid: the first oxazolidinone antimicrobial. Ann Intern Med 2003;138:135–42.

[42] Moellering RC, Jr. Current treatment options for community-acquired methicillin-resistant *Staphylococcus aureus* infection. Clin Infect Dis 2008;46:1032–7.

[43] Cosgrove SE, Fowler VG, Jr. Management of methicillin-resistant *Staphylococcus aureus* bacteremia. Clin Infect Dis 2008;46 Suppl 5:S386–93.

[44] Micek ST. Alternatives to vancomycin for the treatment of methicillin-resistant *Staphylococcus aureus* infections. Clin Infect Dis 2007;45 Suppl 3:S184–90.

[45] Mendes RE, Sader HS, Deshpande L, Jones RN. Antimicrobial activity of tigecycline against community-acquired methicillin-resistant *Staphylococcus aureus* isolates recovered from North American medical centers. Diagn Microbiol Infect Dis 2008;60:433–6.

[46] Stryjewski ME, Chambers HF. Skin and soft-tissue infections caused by community-acquired methicillin-resistant *Staphylococcus aureus*. Clin Infect Dis 2008;46 Suppl 5:S368–77.

[47] Lentino JR, Narita M, Yu VL. New antimicrobial agents as therapy for resistant gram-positive cocci. Eur J Clin Microbiol Infect Dis 2008;27:3–15.

[48] Burkhalter F, Clemenger M, Haddoub SS, McGrory J, Hisole N, Brown E. Pseudomonas exit-site infection: treatment outcomes with topical gentamicin in addition to systemic antibiotics. Clin Kidney J 2015;8:781–4.

[49] Jogi R, Tyring SK. Therapy of nontuberculous mycobacterial infections. Dermatol Ther 2004;17:491–8.

Chapter 7

# Infectious Complications in Peritoneal Dialysis: The Spectrum of Causative Organisms and Recommended Treatment Options

Daniel Kitterer, Joerg Latus, M. Dominik Alscher and
Martin Kimmel

Additional information is available at the end of the chapter

http://dx.doi.org/10.5772/64005

**Abstract**

Peritoneal dialysis (PD) has become a real alternative to hemodialysis (HD) in recent decades, with comparable survival rates, lower costs, and improved patient quality of life. Nevertheless, PD-related infections, including peritonitis, exit-site infections (ESI), and tunnel infections, are important complications, resulting in significant morbidity and a 3.5–10.0% risk of death. Patients with peritonitis usually present with cloudy PD-fluid and abdominal pain; however, PD-associated peritonitis should always be included in differential diagnosis of PD patients with abdominal pain. The most common causative organisms for PD-associated peritonitis are gram-positive bacteria; however, gram-negative species are clinically important, due to the antibiotic resistance. The selection of empiric antibiotics depends on the center-specific distribution of microorganisms and antimicrobial susceptibility profiles. Typically, a first-generation cephalosporin is used in combination with broad gram-negative coverage (e.g., aminoglycoside, ceftazidime, or cefepime). High levels of methicillin-resistant *Staphylococcus epidermidis* or *Enterococcus* spp. strains require the use of vancomycin in many centers. Furthermore, for patients without clinical improvement after 5 days, or with fungal peritonitis, catheter removal is indicated.

**Keywords:** exit-site infections, tunnel infections, CAPD, peritonitis, infectious complications

## 1. Introduction

Georg Ganter published the first trial of peritoneal dialysis (PD) for treatment of uremia in the early twentieth century [1]. Over the following five decades, the technique was developed and mainly used as a procedure in acute kidney failure (AKI) [2], or rarely for patients with chronic kidney disease (CKD) [2]. In 1978, Popovich et al. described a novel sustainable PD technique, which became known as "continuous ambulatory peritoneal dialysis" (CAPD) [3]. CAPD facilitated the introduction of ambulatory PD and paved the way for the widespread use of this renal replacement therapy [4, 5]. When it was initially introduced, the combined 2-year survival rate of patients undergoing CAPD in Europe was only approximately 30% [6].

Over time PD has developed into a real alternative to hemodialysis (HD) with comparable survival rates, lower costs, and improved quality of life for patients [6–9]. Nevertheless, PD-related infections, including peritonitis, exit-site infections (ESI), and tunnel infections, are important complications, resulting in significant morbidity and a 3.5–10.0% risk of death [10]. Consequently, peritonitis is a leading cause of PD failure, resulting in transfer to HD [10, 11], with the associated reduced quality of life for patients [12] and increased costs to the health system [13]. The incidence of peritonitis decreased substantially with the development of disconnect (twin bag) systems and Y-systems [14, 15]. Nowadays, the incidence of PD-associated peritonitis varies from 0.06 to 1.66 episodes/patient-year depending on the center and country [16].

## 2. Clinical presentation and epidemiology

Patients with peritonitis usually present with cloudy PD-fluid and abdominal pain; however, PD-associated peritonitis should always be included in the differential diagnosis of PD patients with abdominal pain, even if the effluent is clear [17]. Furthermore, cloudy effluent can also be indicative of a different underlying disease [18, 19]. In principle, differential diagnoses of cloudy effluent could include, one the one hand, PD-associated infectious peritonitis (culture positive or culture negative), chemical peritonitis (culture negative), or eosinophilia of the effluent (culture negative); or, on the other hand, rare events like malignancy, chylous effluent, or an error of effluent sampling (e.g., a sample taken from a "dry" abdomen). With the introduction of Y-connectors peritonitis rates declined to around 0.7 episodes/patient year (one episode every 18 months; **Figure 1**) [17]; however, overall episode rates as low as one every 41–52 months (0.29–0.23/year) have been reported [15, 20, 21] and ISPD-guidelines recommend that every PD program should monitor infection rates annually at minimum [17]. Definitions and terminology describing PD-associated peritonitis episodes are provided in **Table 1**.

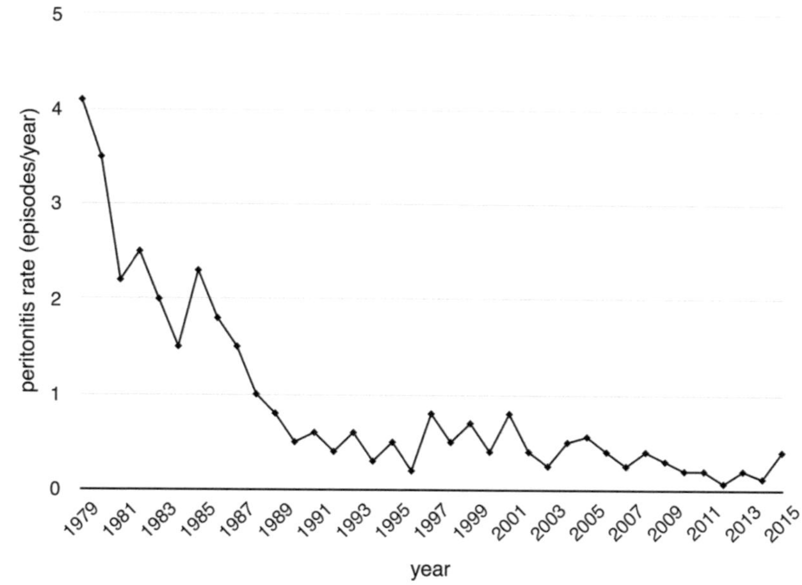


**Figure 1.** Decreasing peritonitis rates over recent decades. The International Society for Peritoneal Dialysis (ISPD) recommended a goal peritonitis rate of 0.7 per patient year.

| Term | Definition |
|---|---|
| Peritonitis | At least two of the criteria*: abdominal pain, effluent with WBC >100/μL (after a dwell time of at least 2 h) and ≥50% polymorphonuclear neutrophilic cells, positive effluent cultures |
| Exit-site infection | Purulent drainage from the exit site. Erythema may or may not represent exit-site infection |
| Tunnel infection | Sonographic evidence of fluid collection (sonolucent zone around the catheter) with or without involvement of the proximal cuff (often clinically occult) |
| Catheter-related peritonitis | Peritonitis in combination with an exit-site or tunnel infection with the same organism, or one site sterile |
| Recurrent peritonitis | An episode that occurs within 4 weeks of completion of therapy for a prior episode but with a different organism |
| Relapsing peritonitis | An episode that occurs within 4 weeks of completion of therapy for a prior episode with the same organism or one sterile episode |
| Repeating peritonitis | An episode that occurs more than 4 weeks after completion of therapy for a prior episode with the same organism |
| Refractory peritonitis | Failure of the effluent to clear after 5-day treatment with appropriate antibiotics |

Adapted with permission from Li et al. [17].

*Peritoneal dialysis patients presenting with cloudy effluent should be presumed to have peritonitis [1].

**Table 1.** Important terminology in PD-associated peritonitis

There are four main routes of entry for peritonitis-causing organisms. The most common path of infection is touch contamination at the time of exchange [22], which is the reason for the predomination of gram-positive strains of skin flora. In some patients with a history of antibiotic use, gram-negative strains can potentially be more numerous on the skin, which may elevate the risk of both gram-negative and fungal peritonitis [23, 24]. In addition, fecal contamination extends the spectrum of causative organisms toward gram-negative strains [25]. The second path of infection is catheter-related (exit-site and/or tunnel infection), and the third is the hematogenous route, although this is very rare [26]. The fourth route of infection in CAPD patients is endogen peritonitis (enteric or gynecological). Common reasons for this type of infection are endoscopic procedures (that require antibiotic prophylaxes [17], possibly abdominal surgery (some centers apply a temporary cessation of PD for 2 weeks for patients undergoing abdominal surgery [27]) and hollow organ or intestinal perforation. Perforation of abdominal organs should always be suspected in peritonitis patients with polymicrobial infections, no response to empiric antibiotic therapy, and a severe clinical course. Abdominal computed tomography (CT) scan should be performed rapidly, although such scans are frequently not diagnostic in this population; hence, early surgical referral is imperative [28, 29]. Peritonitis due to bowel leak (diverticulosis) without intestinal perforation can be managed without surgery; however, an antifungal prophylaxis should be applied [30].

## 3. Diagnostic work up

### 3.1. Cell count

Cloudy effluent should always trigger suspicion of peritonitis. Elevated white cell count (>100/μL), polymorphonuclear (PMN) cells >50%, and positive culture are diagnostic for peritonitis [17]. After catheter implantation, an elevated cell count with eosinophilia, in reaction to the introduction of artificial substances into the body, is common [31, 32] and fungal infections may also rarely be associated with eosinophilia [33, 34].

### 3.2. Culture

Microbiological culture is essential, not only for diagnosis, but also for the choice of anti-infection therapy [17]. Although blood cultures are rarely positive, they should be performed if an additional systemic inflammatory response syndrome is detected. Use of gram stain is controversial but is recommended in the current ISPD-guidelines [17] and can result in early diagnosis of infections [35].

### 3.3. Tunnel ultrasound

Tunnel ultrasound is an important tool to detect fluid collection, particularly in clinically occult tunnel infections [36–38]. This is important, since in patients with exit-site infections, additional tunnel infection increases the risk of catheter-associated peritonitis and loss of catheter [39].

### 3.4. Abdominal imaging

Abdominal imaging is not recommended as standard but must be considered at an early stage when endogenous peritonitis is suspected [28–30].

## 4. Causative pathogens

### 4.1. Gram-positive organisms

The most important causative organisms for PD-associated peritonitis are gram-positive bacteria and, in most centers, coagulase negative staphylococci (CNS) are the most frequent cause of peritonitis [40] (**Figure 2**). Further, *Staphylococcus aureus* can also cause peritonitis, albeit in a smaller proportion of cases; however, infections with this organism should not be underestimated since *S. aureus* peritonitis is a serious complication of PD associated with increased mortality [41, 42]. The majority of recent studies have reported decreases of both CNS and *S. aureus* infections [43, 44] since the introduction of double-bag (twin-bag) and Y-connectors, nasal *S. aureus* screening, and local treatment with mupirocin [45–47]. Otherwise, methicillin-resistant *S. epidermidis* (MRSE) is the most common methicillin-resistant strain [44, 48], whereas methicillin-resistant *S. aureus* (MRSA) is rare [20, 44, 48].

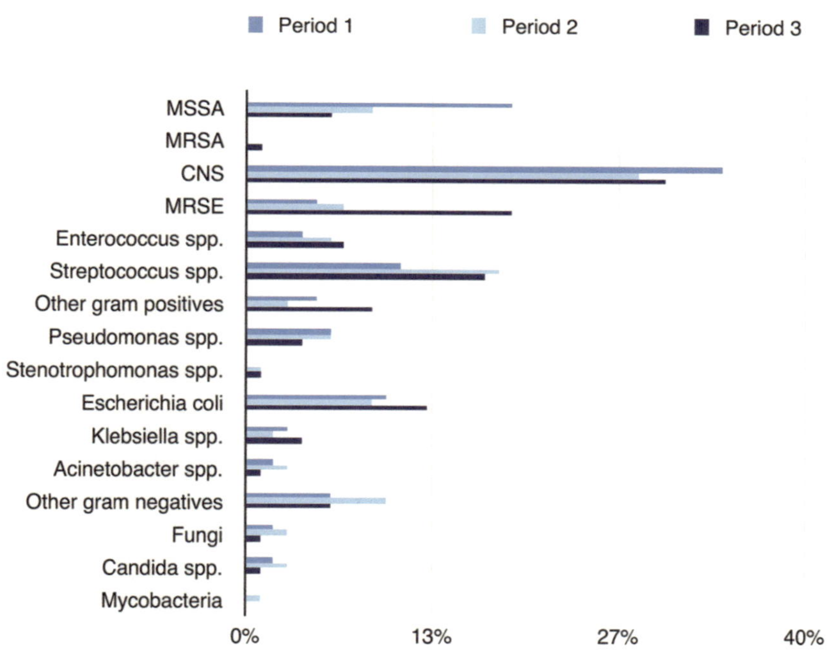


**Figure 2.** Causative pathogens in a single German center [44]. Distribution of organisms in period 1 (1979–1992), period 2 (1993–2003), and period 3 (2004–2014); all variables are expressed as percentages. Abbreviations: MSSA, methicillin-sensitive *S. aureus*; MRSA, methicillin-resistant *S. aureus*; CNS, coagulase-negative staphylococci; MRSE, methicillin-resistant *S. epidermidis*.

### 4.2. Gram-negative organisms

Whether or not gram-negative peritonitis is increasing which remains a topic of discussion and is likely to depend on various local factors [49–51]. The perception that gram-negative peritonitis is increasing may be a consequence of the recent pronounced decrease in gram-positive peritonitis, in the context of gram-negative peritonitis rates that remain constant or are less markedly decreased [44, 52, 53]. Gram-negative organisms are often resistant to antibiotics due to either plasmid encoded beta lactamase (e.g., extended beta lactamase (ESBL) producers) or chromosomally mediated beta-lactamases (e.g., derepressed AmpC beta-lactamase). These organisms are summarized by the acronym SPICE (*Serratia, Pseudomonas/Providencia,* indole-positive *Proteus/Acinetobacter/Morganella, Citrobacter, Enterobacter,* or *Hafnia*) [54, 55]. In addition, third generation cephalosporin-resistant gram-negative (3GCR-GN) rods or ESBL producers [44, 56] are an increasing problem, with ESBL-producing *Escherichia coli* peritonitis associated with worse patient outcomes [57].

### 4.3. Fungal

The majority of fungal peritonitis episodes are associated with prior antibiotic therapy [17]. Fungal prophylaxis during antibiotic therapy should be considered to prevent *Candida* peritonitis in centers with high rates of fungal peritonitis [17], which is a serious complication frequently leading to catheter loss (up to 90% of cases) and an increased risk of death, compared to other organisms [58–61]. Therefore, prompt catheter removal is indicated after identification of fungi by microscopy or culture [17].

### 4.4. Mycobacterium

Mycobacteria-associated peritonitis is rare [44] and, in many patients, only diagnosed after catheter removal from patients with refractory peritonitis.

## 5. Treatment

### 5.1. Initial empiric treatment

The selection of empiric antibiotics will depend on the center-specific distribution of micro-organisms and antimicrobial susceptibility profiles [17]. Typically, a first-generation cephalosporin, such as cefazolin or cephalothin, is used in combination with a drug with broad gram-negative coverage. No significant differences in outcome resulting from treatment with cephalosporins compared to glycopeptides have been reported to date [62]; however, the increasing prevalence of MRSE strains has led to the use of vancomycin in many centers [44]. Moreover, where there is a significant local presence of *Enterococcus* spp., treatment with vancomycin as a first line antibiotic regimen is recommended [63].

Gram-negative coverage can in principle be achieved using an aminoglycoside, ceftazidime, cefepime, or carbapenem [17]. Given the increasing problems due to 3GCR-GN and ESBL resistance, carbapenems are an important class of drugs. In addition, imipenem/cilastatin has similar efficacy in the treatment of PD-associated peritonitis to that of cefazolin plus ceftazidime or netilmicin [64]. However, randomized controlled trials for the use of carbapenems in PD peritonitis are lacking; therefore, routine measurement of blood concentrations should be performed to limit the risk of under- or overdosing [65]. Commonly used anti-infectious drugs for empiric treatment in accordance with the current ISPD-Guidelines are summarized in **Table 2** [17].

| | Intermittent (per exchange, once daily) or continuous (mg/L, all exchanges) application of anti-infective drugs |
|---|---|
| **Gram-positive coverage** | |
| First Generation Cephalosporins[a] | 15 mg/kg/BW i.p. |
| Vancomycin | Loading dose 30 mg/kg/BW, repeated application every 5–7 days adapted to drug levels i.p. |
| Ampicillin | 25 mg/L in each exchange |
| Linezolid | Oral 200–300 mg every day or linezolid 600 mg i.v. twice daily |
| Rifampicin (additional in MRSA peritonitis) | Oral 450 mg every day for <50 kg; 600 mg every day for >50 kg additional to vancomycin |
| **Gram-negative coverage** | |
| Cefepime | 1000 mg i.p. |
| Ceftazidime | 1000–1500 mg i.p. |
| Gentamicin/Tobramicin | 0.6 mg/kg/BW i.p. |
| Ciprofloxacin | Loading dose 50 mg/L, maintenance dose 25 mg/L |
| **Antifungal coverage** | |
| Fluconazole | 200 mg i.p. every 24–48 h |
| Amphotericin | 1.5 mg/L in every bag |
| **Gram-positive and gram-negative coverage** | |
| Imipenem/cilastin | 1 g two times per day i.p. |

All dosage information are adapted with permission from Refs. [17, 66]. Doses of drugs with renal clearance in patients with residual renal function (defined as >100 mL/day urine output) should be empirically increased by 25%.

BW = body weight; IP = intraperitoneal; MRSA = methicillin-resistant *S. aureus*.

[a]Cefazolin or cephalothin.

**Table 2.** Dosing of common anti-infection drugs for empiric, intermittent intraperitoneal first-line regimens in CAPD

### 5.2. Subsequent treatment

#### *5.2.1. CNS and other gram-positive organisms*

In patients for whom microbiological culture results confirm CNS or other gram-positive strains, the current guidelines recommend continuation of empiric gram-positive coverage and endorse adaption of treatment to reflect the local susceptibility profile, if appropriate. Antibiotics targeting gram-negative organisms should simultaneously be stopped [17].

Clinical improvement should be reviewed in a standardized manner, and dialysis effluent cell culture counts repeated on days 3–5. In cases of clinical improvement (symptom-free patient, clear effluent), the antibiotic regimen should be continued for 14 days. It is important to be vigilant for exit-site infections, occult tunnel-infections and intra-abdominal abscesses. Furthermore, potential catheter colonization should be assessed [17].

In general, therapy should continue for 14 days; however, for patients with catheter infection, therapy should be prolonged to 14–21 days and catheter removal considered [17]. An alternative approach is for treatment to be continued for 1 week after cultures become negative and cell counts less than 100 cells/L are reached [67].

In the absence of clinical improvement (persisting symptoms, cloudy effluent), patient samples should be re-cultured and biofilm involvement considered. If no clinical improvement is achieved after 5 days treatment with appropriate antibiotics, the catheter must be removed [17, 19].

#### *5.2.2. Enterococcus/Streptococcus*

In the case of cultures positive for *Enterococcus* spp. or *Streptococcus* spp., the empiric antibiotic regime should alternate with continuous application of ampicillin at 125 mg/L to each bag. Cephalosporins for gram-negative coverage must be stopped and the use of an aminoglycoside for *Enterococcus* treatment considered. Furthermore, it is important to note that ampicillin and aminoglycosides should not be mixed together in the same solution bag. In cases, resistant to ampicillin, vancomycin should be administered.

If vancomycin-resistant *Enterococcus* (VRE) emerges, a streptogramin antibiotic (quinupristin/dalfopristin), daptomycin, or linezolid must be administered, although the choice of therapy should always be guided by local susceptibility profiles. As already explained, the choice of further treatment approach depends on clinical improvement.

Therapy for *Streptococcus* spp.-associated peritonitis is the same as that for patients with *Enterococcus* spp.; however, the therapy durations differ, at 14 and 21 days for *Streptococcus* spp. and *Enterococcus* spp., respectively [17].

#### *5.2.3. S. aureus*

In proven *S. aureus* peritonitis, the empiric gram-positive antibiotic regimen should be continued in accordance with local susceptibility profiles. If there is evidence for vancomycin-resistant *S. aureus*, linezolid, daptomycin, or quinupristin/dalfopristin should be used [17]. Gram-negative coverage should be stopped, and the exit-site closely evaluated.

In the rare cases where a methicillin-resistant strain is detected, the antibiotic regime should be adjusted to a glycopeptide antibiotic (vancomycin or teicoplanin); in addition, rifampin (600 mg/day orally in a single or split dose) can be administered for 5–7 days.

As mentioned above, therapy should then be customized depending on clinical improvement. For *S. aureus*, therapy duration is 21 days. In *S. aureus* peritonitis linked to catheter infection, a refractory infection must be suspected and catheter removal should be considered. If the catheter is removed, a period of 3 weeks must be observed before reinitiation of PD [17].

### 5.3. Culture negative

If first culture is negative on days 1 and 2, empiric therapy should be continued and dialysis effluent cell count and cultures repeated on day 3. If the patient improves clinically, therapy should be continued for 14 days. In patients without clinical improvement, fungi-associated peritonitis should be considered and special culture techniques for unusual causes (e.g., viral, mycoplasma, mycobacteria, *Legionella*) applied [17]. If microbial detection is achieved, the specific anti-infection therapy should be adjusted to the particular microorganism.

If the culture remains negative and no clinical improvement is achieved, the catheter must be removed. In this case, anti-infection therapy should be continued for at least 14 days after catheter removal [17].

#### *5.3.1. Pseudomonas spp.*

If culture indicates *Pseudomonas* spp., it is important to differentiate between peritonitis with catheter infection and peritonitis without catheter infection.

In patients with underlying catheter infection and *Pseudomonas* peritonitis, the catheter must be removed and antibiotic therapy should be continued for at least 14 days. The timing of resumption of peritoneal dialysis may be modified depending on clinical course [17]. If no evidence for exit-site infection or tunnel infection is present, two different antibiotic substances (e.g., *Pseudomonas* spp. effective cephalosporin, aminoglycoside, quinolone, or piperacillin) should be applied. Clinical improvement, dialysis effluent cell counts, and cultures should be assessed on days 3–5.

If patients recover, therapy should continue for at least 21 days. In patients without signs of clinical improvement after 5 days, the catheter should be removed [17].

#### *5.3.2. Single gram-negative organism*

In patients with proven single gram-negative peritonitis, *Stenotrophomonas* must be distinguished from other gram-negative species (*E. coli, Proteus, Klebsiella*, etc.). *Stenotrophomonas*-associated peritonitis must be treated similarly to *Pseudomonas*-associated peritonitis, using two different antibiotics with different mechanisms of action, based on the local sensitivity pattern (e.g., oral trimethoprim/sulfamethoxazole in combination with quinolones). Again, clinical improvement should be reviewed and dialysis effluent cell count cultures repeated on days 3–5. In cases of clinical improvement, therapy can be resumed after a duration of 21–28 days [17], otherwise the catheter must be removed.

In gram-negative non-*Stenotrophomonas*-associated peritonitis, empiric therapy should be adjusted to account for local susceptibility profiles. Cephalosporins, aminoglycosides, or carbapenems may be indicated. Gram-positive coverage should be stopped. In cases of clinical improvement, antibiotic therapy should be continued for 14–21 days. If no clinical improvement can be achieved, the catheter must be removed [17].

#### *5.3.3. Polymicrobial peritonitis*

In patients with polymicrobial peritonitis, multiple gram-negative organisms or mixed gram-negative/gram-positive organisms must be differentiated from multiple gram-positive organisms which indicate touch contamination or catheter infection.

Mixed gram-negative/gram-positive infections or multiple gram-negative-infections should always raise suspicion of endogenous peritonitis. Anti-infection therapy should be changed to metronidazole in combination with ampicillin, ceftazidime, or aminoglycosides. Further, an abdominal CT-scan is suggested and urgent surgical assessment is required. In patients with "surgical" peritonitis, the catheter must be removed and anti-infection therapy should be continued for 14 days [17].

In patients with polymicrobial gram-positive peritonitis, without diagnosis of catheter infection, anti-infection therapy adapted to local susceptibility profiles should be continued for at least 21 days. In patients with catheter infection, the catheter should be removed [17].

### 5.4. Other indications for catheter removal

Other indications for catheter removal are refractory infections or relapsing episodes. Further, in catheter-related infections with or without formation of biofilms, catheter removal should be considered and fungal infections always require catheter removal [68]. In *Pseudomonas aeruginosa*-associated peritonitis, prompt catheter removal and a double *P. aeruginosa* effective antibiotic regimen should be followed [69].

## 6. Prevention

### 6.1. "Single shot" antibiotic treatment at catheter implantation

A systematic Cochrane review investigated prophylactic antibiotic use at catheter insertion versus no antibiotic application at implantation in four trials, including 355 patients. The authors concluded that the use of perioperative intravenous antibiotic prophylaxis significantly decreased the risk of early peritonitis compared to no treatment [70]. Consistent with these findings, an ISPD-position statement recommended that prophylaxis with a first generation cephalosporin (e.g., cefazolin) or vancomycin, and prophylaxis at catheter placement, should be considered in each PD program, taking into consideration any emerging local resistance to vancomycin [16].

### 6.2. Peritoneal access and the role of catheter design

Two large meta-analyses, including 859 patients, confirmed that the risk for PD-associated infections did not differ significantly with various catheter designs [71, 72]. Therefore, the current ISP-Guidelines recommend no specific catheter design to prevent peritonitis [16]. Regarding peritoneal access, no significant differences in the rate of peritonitis or exit-site infections were observed when laparoscopy versus standard laparotomy, or subcutaneous catheter insertion was used [72–75]. However, a minimally invasive approach results in higher 1-year catheter survival and less frequent catheter migration, compared to laparotomy, according to a recent meta-analysis [72].

### 6.3. Eradication of *S. aureus*

A 1990 study by Luzar et al. demonstrating that nasal carriers of *S. aureus* have an increased risk of ESI and peritonitis [76] underlies the implementation of *S. aureus* screening in some PD programs. A large meta-analysis, including a total of 14 studies, 1233 enrolled patients and a similarly large control group, showed that mupirocin application was associated with a significantly lower risk of ESI and peritonitis [77]. However, no randomized control trials (RCTs) comparing the effectiveness of applying mupirocin to the catheter exit site against placebo have been conducted to date, although Bernardini et al. investigated the topical application of gentamicin versus mupirocin in 133 patients in an RCT [78]. The authors showed an advantage for gentamicin versus mupirocin for reducing catheter infection and peritonitis rates [78]; however, the long-term application of gentamicin may results in gentamicin-resistant organisms [79], which can potentially complicate peritonitis. Regardless, the ISP recommends topical application of antibiotic to the catheter exit-site in all patients [16].

### 6.4. Antimycotic prophylaxis in PD patients receiving antibiotics

Patients who receive prolonged or repeated antibiotics are at increased risk of developing fungal peritonitis [17]. Two RCTs compared antifungal prophylaxis in PD patients receiving antibiotic therapy [80, 81]. Lo et al. found an advantage of Nystatin as an antifungal prophylaxis during any antibiotic therapy; however, the trial was conducted in a population with a high incidence of fungal peritonitis. Restrepo et al. investigated 420 patients who received antibiotics for PD-associated complications and compared fluconazol as prophylaxis versus placebo. Both studies found that prophylaxis reduced the relative risk of fungal peritonitis. The ISPD working group recommends that each PD program should monitor their history of fungal peritonitis and decide if an antifungal with antibiotic protocol would be beneficial, particularly for patients taking prolonged or frequent courses of antibiotics [16, 17].

## Author details

Daniel Kitterer, Joerg Latus, M. Dominik Alscher and Martin Kimmel

*Address all correspondence to: martin.kimmel@rbk.de

Department of Internal Medicine, Division of General Internal Medicine and Nephrology, Robert-Bosch Hospital, Stuttgart, Germany

## References

[1] Ganter G. Über die Beseitigung giftiger Stoffe aus dem Blut durch Dialyse. Munch Med Wschr. 1923;70:1478–80.

[2] Grollman A, Turner LB, Mc LJ. Intermittent peritoneal lavage in nephrectomized dogs and its application to the human being. AMA Arch Intern Med. 1951;87(3):379–90.

[3] Popovich RP, Moncrief JW, Nolph KD, Ghods AJ, Twardowski ZJ, Pyle WK. Continuous ambulatory peritoneal dialysis. Ann Intern Med. 1978;88(4):449–56.

[4] Oreopoulos DG, Robson M, Izatt S, Clayton S, deVeber GA. A simple and safe technique for continuous ambulatory peritoneal dialysis (CAPD). Trans Am Soc Artif Intern Organs. 1978;24:484–9.

[5] Nolph KD, Sorkin M, Rubin J, Arfania D, Prowant B, Fruto L, et al. Continuous ambulatory peritoneal dialysis: three-year experience at one center. Ann Intern Med. 1980;92(5):609–13.

[6] Jacobs C, Broyer M, Brunner FP, Brynger H, Donckerwolcke RA, Kramer P, et al. Combined report on regular dialysis and transplantation in Europe, XI, 1980. Proc Eur Dial Transplant Assoc. 1981;18:4–58.

[7] Lee CC, Sun CY, Wu MS. Long-term modality-related mortality analysis in incident dialysis patients. Perit Dial Int. 2009;29(2):182–90.

[8] Ginieri-Coccossis M, Theofilou P, Synodinou C, Tomaras V, Soldatos C. Quality of life, mental health and health beliefs in haemodialysis and peritoneal dialysis patients: investigating differences in early and later years of current treatment. BMC Nephrol. 2008;9:14.

[9] Salonen T, Reina T, Oksa H, Sintonen H, Pasternack A. Cost analysis of renal replacement therapies in Finland. Am J Kidney Dis. 2003;42(6):1228–38.

[10] Mujais S. Microbiology and outcomes of peritonitis in North America. Kidney Int Suppl. 2006(103):S55–62.

[11] Afolalu B, Troidle L, Osayimwen O, Bhargava J, Kitsen J, Finkelstein FO. Technique failure and center size in a large cohort of peritoneal dialysis patients in a defined geographic area. Perit Dial Int. 2009;29(3):292–6.

[12] Kutner NG, Zhang R, Barnhart H, Collins AJ. Health status and quality of life reported by incident patients after 1 year on haemodialysis or peritoneal dialysis. Nephrol Dial Transplant. 2005;20(10):2159–67.

[13] Lo WK. Peritoneal dialysis utilization and outcome: what are we facing? Perit Dial Int. 2007;27(Suppl 2):S42–7.

[14] Peritonitis in continuous ambulatory peritoneal dialysis (CAPD): a multi-centre randomized clinical trial comparing the Y connector disinfectant system to standard systems. Canadian CAPD Clinical Trials Group. Perit Dial Int. 1989;9(3):159–63.

[15] Li PK, Law MC, Chow KM, Chan WK, Szeto CC, Cheng YL, et al. Comparison of clinical outcome and ease of handling in two double-bag systems in continuous ambulatory peritoneal dialysis: a prospective, randomized, controlled, multicenter study. Am J Kidney Dis. 2002;40(2):373–80.

[16] Piraino B, Bernardini J, Brown E, Figueiredo A, Johnson DW, Lye WC, et al. ISPD position statement on reducing the risks of peritoneal dialysis-related infections. Perit Dial Int. 2011;31(6):614–30.

[17] Li PK, Szeto CC, Piraino B, Bernardini J, Figueiredo AE, Gupta A, et al. Peritoneal dialysis-related infections recommendations: 2010 update. Perit Dial Int. 2010;30(4): 393–423.

[18] Rocklin MA, Teitelbaum I. Noninfectious causes of cloudy peritoneal dialysate. Semin Dial. 2001;14(1):37–40.

[19] Ekart R, Horvat M, Kozelj M, Balon BP, Bevc S, Hojs R. Gangrenous appendicitis presenting as acute abdominal pain in a patient on automated peritoneal dialysis: a case report. J Med Case Rep. 2012;6:309.

[20] Kim DK, Yoo TH, Ryu DR, Xu ZG, Kim HJ, Choi KH, et al. Changes in causative organisms and their antimicrobial susceptibilities in CAPD peritonitis: a single center's experience over one decade. Perit Dial Int. 2004;24(5):424–32.

[21] Hasegawa T, Nakai S, Moriishi M, Ito Y, Itami N, Masakane I, et al. Peritoneal dialysis registry with 2012 survey report. Ther Apher Dial. 2015;19(6):529–39.

[22] von Graevenitz A, Amsterdam D. Microbiological aspects of peritonitis associated with continuous ambulatory peritoneal dialysis. Clin Microbiol Rev. 1992;5(1):36–48.

[23] Goldie SJ, Kiernan-Tridle L, Torres C, Gorban-Brennan N, Dunne D, Kliger AS, et al. Fungal peritonitis in a large chronic peritoneal dialysis population: a report of 55 episodes. Am J Kidney Dis. 1996;28(1):86–91.

[24] Szeto CC, Chow KM, Leung CB, Wong TY, Wu AK, Wang AY, et al. Clinical course of peritonitis due to *Pseudomonas* species complicating peritoneal dialysis: a review of 104 cases. Kidney Int. 2001;59(6):2309–15.

[25] Prasad N, Gupta A, Sharma RK, Prasad KN, Gulati S, Sharma AP. Outcome of gram-positive and gram-negative peritonitis in patients on continuous ambulatory peritoneal dialysis: a single-center experience. Perit Dial Int. 2003;23(Suppl 2):S144–7.

[26] Selgas R, Munoz J, Aquella A, Huarte E, Fonseca E, Escuin F, et al. Mycobacterium chelonei peritonitis due to hematogenous dissemination in a continuous ambulatory peritoneal dialysis patient. Am J Kidney Dis. 1987;10(2):144–6.

[27] Goel S, Ribby KJ, Kathuria P, Khanna R. Temporary stoppage of peritoneal dialysis when laparoscopic procedures are performed on patients undergoing CAPD/CCPD: a change in policy. Adv Perit Dial. 1998;14:80–2.

[28] Carmeci C, Muldowney W, Mazbar SA, Bloom R. Emergency laparotomy in patients on continuous ambulatory peritoneal dialysis. Am Surg. 2001;67(7):615–8.

[29] Miller GV, Bhandari S, Brownjohn AM, Turney JH, Benson EA. 'Surgical' peritonitis in the CAPD patient. Ann R Coll Surg Engl. 1998;80(1):36–9.

[30] Suh H, Wadhwa NK, Cabralda T, Sorrento J. Endogenous peritonitis and related outcome in peritoneal dialysis patients. Adv Perit Dial. 1996;12:192–5.

[31] Chan MK, Chow L, Lam SS, Jones B. Peritoneal eosinophilia in patients on continuous ambulatory peritoneal dialysis: a prospective study. Am J Kidney Dis. 1988;11(2):180–3.

[32] Fontan MP, Rodriguez-Carmona A, Galed I, Iglesias P, Villaverde P, Garcia-Ureta E. Incidence and significance of peritoneal eosinophilia during peritoneal dialysis-related peritonitis. Perit Dial Int. 2003;23(5):460–4.

[33] Lee SH, Huang TS. Persistent eosinophilic peritonitis associated with fungal infection cured by resection of external Tenckhoff catheter: a case report. Perit Dial Int. 1997;17(4): 397–9.

[34] Sridhar R, Thornley-Brown D, Kant KS. Peritonitis due to Aspergillus niger: diagnostic importance of peritoneal eosinophilia. Perit Dial Int. 1990;10(1):100–1.

[35] Lee CC, Sun CY, Chang KC, Wu MS. Positive dialysate gram stain predicts outcome of empirical antibiotic therapy for peritoneal dialysis-associated peritonitis. Ther Apher Dial. 2010;14(2):201–8.

[36] Kwan TH, Tong MK, Siu YP, Leung KT, Luk SH, Cheung YK. Ultrasonography in the management of exit site infections in peritoneal dialysis patients. Nephrology (Carlton). 2004;9(6):348–52.

[37] Korzets Z, Erdberg A, Golan E, Ben-Chitrit S, Verner M, Rathaus V, et al. Frequent involvement of the internal cuff segment in CAPD peritonitis and exit-site infection – an ultrasound study. Nephrol Dial Transplant. 1996;11(2):336–9.

[38] Karahan OI, Taskapan H, Yikilmaz A, Oymak O, Utas C. Ultrasound evaluation of peritoneal catheter tunnel in catheter related infections in CAPD. Int Urol Nephrol. 2005;37(2):363–6.

[39] Domico J, Warman M, Jaykamur S, Sorkin MI. Is ultrasonography useful in predicting catheter loss? Adv Perit Dial. 1993;9:231–2.

[40] Camargo CH, Cunha Mde L, Caramori JC, Mondelli AL, Montelli AC, Barretti P. Peritoneal dialysis-related peritonitis due to coagulase-negative Staphylococcus: a review of 115 cases in a Brazilian center. Clin J Am Soc Nephrol. 2014;9(6):1074–81.

[41] Szeto CC, Chow KM, Kwan BC, Law MC, Chung KY, Yu S, et al. *Staphylococcus aureus* peritonitis complicates peritoneal dialysis: review of 245 consecutive cases. Clin J Am Soc Nephrol. 2007;2(2):245–51.

[42] Barretti P, Moraes TM, Camargo CH, Caramori JC, Mondelli AL, Montelli AC, et al. Peritoneal dialysis-related peritonitis due to *Staphylococcus aureus*: a single-center experience over 15 years. PLoS One. 2012;7(2):e31780.

[43] Kavanagh D, Prescott GJ, Mactier RA. Peritoneal dialysis-associated peritonitis in Scotland (1999–2002). Nephrol Dial Transplant. 2004;19(10):2584–91.

[44] Kitterer D, Latus J, Pohlmann C, Alscher MD, Kimmel M. Microbiological surveillance of peritoneal dialysis associated peritonitis: antimicrobial susceptibility profiles of a referral center in GERMANY over 32 years. PLoS One. 2015;10(9):e0135969.

[45] Bazzato G, Coli U, Landini S, Fracasso A, Morachiello P, Righetto F, et al. The double bag system for CAPD reduces the peritonitis rate. Trans Am Soc Artif Intern Organs. 1984;30:690–2.

[46] Daly C, Campbell M, Cody J, Grant A, Donaldson C, Vale L, et al. Double bag or Y-set versus standard transfer systems for continuous ambulatory peritoneal dialysis in end-stage renal disease. Cochrane Database Syst Rev. 2001(2):CD003078.

[47] Nasal mupirocin prevents *Staphylococcus aureus* exit-site infection during peritoneal dialysis. Mupirocin Study Group. J Am Soc Nephrol. 1996;7(11):2403–8.

[48] Holley JL, Bernardini J, Johnston JR, Piraino B. Methicillin-resistant staphylococcal infections in an outpatient peritoneal dialysis program. Am J Kidney Dis. 1990;16(2): 142–6.

[49] Brown F, Gulyani A, McDonald S, Hurst K.; Peritoneal Dialysis Anzdata Registry 2012 Report (2013). Available from: http://www.anzdata.org.au/anzdata/AnzdataReport/35thReport/2012c06_peritoneal_v3.pdf.

[50] Rocha A, Rodrigues A, Teixeira L, Carvalho MJ, Mendonca D, Cabrita A. Temporal trends in peritonitis rates, microbiology and outcomes: the major clinical complication of peritoneal dialysis. Blood Purif. 2012;33(4):284–91.

[51] Ozisik L, Ozdemir FN, Tanriover MD. The changing trends of peritoneal dialysis related peritonitis and novel risk factors. Ren Fail. 2015;37(6):1027–32.

[52] Han SH, Lee SC, Ahn SV, Lee JE, Choi HY, Kim BS, et al. Improving outcome of CAPD: twenty-five years' experience in a single Korean center. Perit Dial Int. 2007;27(4):432–40.

[53] van Esch S, Krediet RT, Struijk DG. 32 years' experience of peritoneal dialysis-related peritonitis in a university hospital. Perit Dial Int. 2014;34(2):162–70.

[54] Friedman O, Jassal SV, Bargman JM. *Acinetobacter* peritoneal dialysis peritonitis: description and relation to the SPICE family of organisms. Perit Dial Int. 2008;28(2): 195–7.

[55] Chao CT, Lee SY, Yang WS, Chen HW, Fang CC, Yen CJ, et al. *Acinetobacter* peritoneal dialysis peritonitis: a changing landscape over time. PLoS One. 2014;9(10):e110315.

[56] Feng X, Yang X, Yi C, Guo Q, Mao H, Jiang Z, et al. *Escherichia coli* Peritonitis in peritoneal dialysis: the prevalence, antibiotic resistance and clinical outcomes in a South China dialysis center. Perit Dial Int. 2014;34(3):308–16.

[57] Yip T, Tse KC, Lam MF, Tang S, Li FK, Choy BY, et al. Risk factors and outcomes of extended-spectrum beta-lactamase-producing *E. coli* peritonitis in CAPD patients. Perit Dial Int. 2006;26(2):191–7.

[58] Miles R, Hawley CM, McDonald SP, Brown FG, Rosman JB, Wiggins KJ, et al. Predictors and outcomes of fungal peritonitis in peritoneal dialysis patients. Kidney Int. 2009;76(6):622–8.

[59] Chan TM, Chan CY, Cheng SW, Lo WK, Lo CY, Cheng IK. Treatment of fungal peritonitis complicating continuous ambulatory peritoneal dialysis with oral fluconazole: a series of 21 patients. Nephrol Dial Transplant. 1994;9(5):539–42.

[60] Chen P, Johnson P, Sommer T, Jentsch S, Hochstrasser M. Multiple ubiquitin-conjugating enzymes participate in the in vivo degradation of the yeast MAT alpha 2 repressor. Cell. 1993;74(2):357–69.

[61] Oh SH, Conley SB, Rose GM, Rosenblum M, Kohl S, Pickering LK. Fungal peritonitis in children undergoing peritoneal dialysis. Pediatr Infect Dis. 1985;4(1):62–6.

[62] Khairullah Q, Provenzano R, Tayeb J, Ahmad A, Balakrishnan R, Morrison L. Comparison of vancomycin versus cefazolin as initial therapy for peritonitis in peritoneal dialysis patients. Perit Dial Int. 2002;22(3):339–44.

[63] Edey M, Hawley CM, McDonald SP, Brown FG, Rosman JB, Wiggins KJ, et al. Enterococcal peritonitis in Australian peritoneal dialysis patients: predictors, treatment and outcomes in 116 cases. Nephrol Dial Transplant. 2010;25(4):1272–8.

[64] Leung CB, Szeto CC, Chow KM, Kwan BC, Wang AY, Lui SF, et al. Cefazolin plus ceftazidime versus imipenem/cilastatin monotherapy for treatment of CAPD peritonitis—randomized controlled trial. Perit Dial Int. 2004;24(5):440–6.

[65] Vlaar PJ, van Hulst M, Benne CA, Janssen WM. Intraperitoneal compared with intravenous meropenem for peritoneal dialysis-related peritonitis. Perit Dial Int. 2013;33(6):708–9.

[66] Yang JW, Kim YS, Choi SO, Han BG. Successful use of intravenous linezolid in CAPD patient with vancomycin-resistant enterococcal peritonitis. Perit Dial Int. 2011;31(2): 209–10.

[67] Boeschoten EW, Rietra PJ, Krediet RT, Visser MJ, Arisz L. CAPD peritonitis: a prospective randomized trial of oral versus intraperitoneal treatment with cephradine. J Antimicrob Chemother. 1985;16(6):789–97.

[68] Levallois J, Nadeau-Fredette AC, Labbe AC, Laverdiere M, Ouimet D, Vallee M. Ten-year experience with fungal peritonitis in peritoneal dialysis patients: antifungal susceptibility patterns in a North-American center. Int J Infect Dis. 2012;16(1):e41–3.

[69] Siva B, Hawley CM, McDonald SP, Brown FG, Rosman JB, Wiggins KJ, et al. *Pseudomonas* peritonitis in Australia: predictors, treatment, and outcomes in 191 cases. Clin J Am Soc Nephrol. 2009;4(5):957–64.

[70] Strippoli GF, Tong A, Johnson D, Schena FP, Craig JC. Antimicrobial agents for preventing peritonitis in peritoneal dialysis patients. Cochrane Database Syst Rev. 2004(4):CD004679.

[71] Strippoli GF, Tong A, Johnson D, Schena FP, Craig JC. Catheter type, placement and insertion techniques for preventing peritonitis in peritoneal dialysis patients. Cochrane Database Syst Rev. 2004(4):CD004680.

[72] Hagen SM, Lafranca JA, JN IJ, Dor FJ. A systematic review and meta-analysis of the influence of peritoneal dialysis catheter type on complication rate and catheter survival. Kidney Int. 2014;85(4):920–32.

[73] Tsimoyiannis EC, Siakas P, Glantzounis G, Toli C, Sferopoulos G, Pappas M, et al. Laparoscopic placement of the Tenckhoff catheter for peritoneal dialysis. Surg Laparosc Endosc Percutan Tech. 2000;10(4):218–21.

[74] Gadallah MF, Pervez A, el-Shahawy MA, Sorrells D, Zibari G, McDonald J, et al. Peritoneoscopic versus surgical placement of peritoneal dialysis catheters: a prospective randomized study on outcome. Am J Kidney Dis. 1999;33(1):118–22.

[75] Wright MJ, Bel'eed K, Johnson BF, Eadington DW, Sellars L, Farr MJ. Randomized prospective comparison of laparoscopic and open peritoneal dialysis catheter insertion. Perit Dial Int. 1999;19(4):372–5.

[76] Luzar MA, Coles GA, Faller B, Slingeneyer A, Dah GD, Briat C, et al. *Staphylococcus aureus* nasal carriage and infection in patients on continuous ambulatory peritoneal dialysis. N Engl J Med. 1990;322(8):505–9.

[77] Xu G, Tu W, Xu C. Mupirocin for preventing exit-site infection and peritonitis in patients undergoing peritoneal dialysis. Nephrol Dial Transplant. 2010;25(2):587–92.

[78] Bernardini J, Bender F, Florio T, Sloand J, Palmmontalbano L, Fried L, et al. Randomized, double-blind trial of antibiotic exit site cream for prevention of exit site infection in peritoneal dialysis patients. J Am Soc Nephrol. 2005;16(2):539–45.

[79] Pierce DA, Williamson JC, Mauck VS, Russell GB, Palavecino E, Burkart JM. The effect on peritoneal dialysis pathogens of changing topical antibiotic prophylaxis. Perit Dial Int. 2012;32(5):525–30.

[80] Lo WK, Chan CY, Cheng SW, Poon JF, Chan DT, Cheng IK. A prospective randomized control study of oral nystatin prophylaxis for *Candida* peritonitis complicating continuous ambulatory peritoneal dialysis. Am J Kidney Dis. 1996;28(4):549–52.

[81] Restrepo C, Chacon J, Manjarres G. Fungal peritonitis in peritoneal dialysis patients: successful prophylaxis with fluconazole, as demonstrated by prospective randomized control trial. Perit Dial Int. 2010;30(6):619–25.

# Chapter 8

# Is Peritoneal Dialysis a Suitable Method of Renal Replacement Therapy in Acute Kidney Injury?

Damir Rebić and Vedad Herenda

Additional information is available at the end of the chapter

http://dx.doi.org/10.5772/64668

**Abstract**

*Research focus*: The role of peritoneal dialysis (PD) in the management of acute kidney injury (AKI) is not well defined, although it remains frequently used, especially in low-resource settings. A review was performed to ascertain its suitability as the "first choice" in AKI patient treatment and to compare PD with extracorporeal blood purification (EBP), such as hemodialysis (HD). *Research methods used*: Design, setting, participants, and measurements of MEDLINE, CINAHL, and Central Register of Controlled Trials were searched. The review selected eligible adult population studies on PD in the setting of AKI. *Results/findings of the research*: This paper suggests that PD should be considered as a valuable method for AKI since it offers several advantages over HD, such as technical simplicity, no extracorporeal circuit, and no bleeding risk. It offers good cardiovascular tolerance and less cardiovascular instability, thus reducing kidney aggression by ischemia and hydroelectrolytic imbalance. *Main conclusions and recommendations*: Finally, not only in developing countries but also in developed countries, PD is relatively simple and inexpensive and is more widely used. Various techniques of PD have been developed, and these have been adapted for use in AKI. There is currently no evidence to suggest significant differences in mortality between PD and HD in AKI. There is a need for further good-quality evidence in this important area.

**Keywords:** acute peritoneal dialysis, acute kidney injury, extracorporeal blood purification, suitability, renal recovery

## 1. Introduction

Peritoneal dialysis (PD) was initially used in the 1920s to treat acute kidney injury (AKI), but it was not until 1946 that it was first described in saving the life of a patient. In the 1970s, acute

PD was widely accepted for AKI treatment, but its practice declined in favor of hemodialysis (HD). It is frequently used in developing countries because of its lower cost and minimal infrastructural requirements. The role of peritoneal dialysis in the regimen of patients with AKI is not well defined. In a recent review on the dose of dialysis in AKI, PD was not even mentioned as a potential modality [1].

The use of PD for AKI, then, became somewhat limited and did not receive much attention until 2008. In the year 2008 has rekindled interest in PD for AKI with a series of publications in which they used a randomized trial design. They confirmed efficacy of PD to demonstrate that results with PD are at least as good as those with HD [2, 3].

AKI is defined as an abrupt decline in glomerular filtration rate (GFR) resulting in progressive elevation of plasma urea and creatinine and is an important cause of morbidity and mortality worldwide [4]. AKI is a major cause of morbidity and mortality in critically ill patients and in aging populations. About 30% of patients admitted to intensive care units (ICUs) develop hemodynamic instability, cardiorenal syndrome, and sepsis [5].

The epidemiology of AKI is faintly documented, especially in developing countries. Primarily, this is because of variable definitions of AKI [6]. Nonetheless, it can be safely assumed that AKI is an associated high mortality and morbidity. It is therefore important to continue to evaluate PD as a modality of renal replacement therapy (RRT) in AKI. This is particularly so for centers in countries which often lack the technical support to effectively perform extracorporeal blood purification (EBP). In these settings, PD may be the most practical form of RRT.

## 2. The use of peritoneal dialysis in AKI

Dialysis modalities used in AKI are hemodialysis (HD), continuous renal replacement therapy (CRRT), and acute PD either manually or with automated machines in advanced centers. PD is practiced for AKI treatment mostly due to its cost-effectiveness and the minimal infrastructure required, important considerations in many developing countries. PD is an accessible and effective method for AKI treatment mainly because it's quite simple. At times of major disasters, PD could be a lifesaving therapy. For example, the second most frequent cause of death after direct trauma during disasters is crush injury, and it could be treated with PD [7, 8].

The recent consensus guidelines published by International Society of Peritoneal Dialysis (ISPD) on PD for AKI are an important step in providing RRT uniformly [9, 10]. PD is still an underutilized modality in developed countries for reasons that are unclear, and CRRT is more widely used [11]. However, CRRT requires multiple accesses to bloodstream in critically ill patients, which predisposes them to blood-borne infections and possible circulatory complications. PD is hemodynamically friendly and requires only a single access to the peritoneal cavity, and fluid removal can be smoothly achieved by altering the concentration of glucose in the dialysis fluid. Continuous glucose absorption provides nutritional benefits to the critically ill patient.

The use of PD was associated with a shorter time to renal recovery in the research of Kilonzo et al. [7]. PD is a more physiological and less inflammatory mode of dialysis than HD and better preserves residual renal function [12]. It is likely that the same is true in AKI, although further studies are needed to assess the effect of PD on survival [13]. However, the use of PD for AKI in adults has not attracted much attention from researchers with just few randomized controlled trials in adults in the past 40 years. However, the paucity of literature on PD does not imply that its use is waning. PD is often the only method of supporting a patient with AKI, particularly in developing countries.

### 2.1. Techniques: dosing and adequacy of acute PD

Various techniques (**Table 1**) of peritoneal dialysis have been described in the literature, and these have been adapted for use in AKI. These different techniques are used according to patient requirement and facility preference. The urea clearance is 8–12 mL/min for acute intermittent peritoneal dialysis (AIPD), 15 mL/min for tidal peritoneal dialysis (TPD), and 30–35 mL/min for continuous flow peritoneal dialysis (CFPD) [14].

| Technique | Description |
|---|---|
| Acute intermittent peritoneal dialysis (AIPD) | Most often used in the past. Frequent and short exchanges with volumes 1–2 L and dialysate flows of 2–6 L/h. Each session lasts 16–20 h, usually tri-session per week. The solute clearance is likely inadequate due to its intermittent nature |
| Tidal peritoneal dialysis (TPD) | Typically involves an initial infusion of 3 L of dialysate into the peritoneal cavity. A portion of dialysate, tidal drain volume (usually 1–1.5 L), is drained and replaced with fresh dialysate (tidal fill volume). The reserve volume always remains in the peritoneal cavity throughout the tidal cycle |
| Continuous flow peritoneal dialysis (CFPD) | Inflow and outflow of dialysate occur simultaneously through two access routes. By inflow of 300 mL/min, it is possible to achieve a high-peritoneal urea clearance |
| High-volume peritoneal dialysis (HVPD) | Continuous therapy proposed to increase high small-solute clearances. Frequent exchanges, usually with cycler (18–48 exchanges per 24 h, 2 L per exchange). The total dialysate volume ranges from 36 to 70 L a day |
| Continuous equilibrated peritoneal dialysis (CEPD) | Long dwells of 2–6 h with up to 2 L of dialysate each (similar to CAPD). The clearance of small molecules may be also inadequate, but clearance of middle molecules is possibly higher due to the long dwells |

**Table 1.** Techniques of PD for AKI treatment.

This raises the question, why is the use of PD for AKI declining? The use of PD is precluded in some circumstances, such as after major abdominal surgery or trauma. Patients with AKI are hypercatabolic and require adequate clearance of toxins to avoid complications. Part of the reason for underuse of PD may be related to the perception that PD is not adequate for treatment of AKI. The ultrafiltration (UF) volume could be better controlled with current machines for EBP than with PD. However, published studies report efficient fluid removal and metabolic control in patients on PD. With the decline in the use of PD for AKI worldwide, the clinical experience of the physician as well as the supporting staff in the use of this modality becomes limited due to the lack of exposure.

Recent data from randomized and observational studies on EBP have indicated that, beyond a certain threshold, further increments in dose had no benefits [15, 16]. Low doses and inadequate dialysis contribute to poor outcomes, and augmenting dose may reap increasing benefits until a certain limit is reached. In uremic patients who receive no dialysis, mortality is close to 100%. The probability of survival improves with dialysis. The data on recovery of both the patient and the kidney in those treated with PD are lacking. So far, the dose of dialysis that should be targeted for AKI is unknown.

#### *2.1.1. Clearance of small solutes*

This is most often represented by urea clearance which had been developed for the assessment of chronic dialysis patients, and this model is often applied to AKI as well. However, urea kinetic modelling (UKM) is not held true in an unstable patient and not validated for use in AKI [17, 18]. It continues to be utilized in AKI only due to a lack of alternatives.

To date, there has been very limited data on the effect of dose of PD on AKI. There are no studies which have directly compared various dosing levels in PD and its effect on outcomes.

Studies on EBP [17, 19, 20], which reported dose in terms of $Kt/V_{urea}$, were selected for inference of PD dose in this review even if there are some limitations. The standardized (std)-$Kt/V_{urea}$ minimum target for chronic PD is 1.7 which is lower than weekly std-$Kt/V_{urea}$ of 2.1 in chronic HD.

Patients with AKI are generally catabolic, and adequate clearance of toxins and electrolytes is necessary. It remains to be determined if it is necessary to aim for similar small-solute clearance targets as for HD in the management of AKI.

Inadequate small-solute clearance in dialysis is known to be detrimental. The optimal dose of dialysis for AKI remains uncertain. The minimum dose of peritoneal dialysis that should be achieved according to EBP studies is a std-$Kt/V_{urea}$ of 2.1. It must be emphasized that this is not a fixed dose target for all patients. Higher small-solute clearances may be necessary for patients with more complex catabolic illnesses. But if the small-solute clearance target is met, then clinicians can focus on other aspects of adequacy which may result in improvement in patient outcomes.

#### *2.1.2. Clearance of larger molecules*

The clearance of middle-molecular-weight (MMW) substances is important in certain clinical scenarios such as sepsis-related AKI, where clearance of pro-inflammatory cytokines may attenuate the inflammatory response [16, 21]. There is currently no established method of prescribing dialysis based on middle molecular clearance. No recommendations can be made with regard to any minimum targets of clearances of MMW substances.

### *2.1.3. Other aspects of adequacy*

The removal of uremic toxins is not the sole aim in renal replacement therapy. Fluid status and other homeostatic mechanisms of the kidney are important aspects that encompass dialysis adequacy.

Fluid balance may possibly act as a biomarker of severity in critical illness [22]. A neutral fluid balance has also been shown to improve outcomes in acute lung injury. PD is usually well tolerated with better hemodynamic stability, and it is therefore often recommended as a form of RRT for subgroups such as the elderly or patients with congestive heart failure [23]. Besides removal of uremic toxins, dialysis must also remove fluid and salt from the patient. With a properly functioning PD catheter, exchanges of 2 L of dialysate with 2.5 or 4.25% glucose concentration provide daily fluid removal at the same or greater rate than other regimens without causing hypotension in most patients.

Adequacy of dialysis dose is controversial since many authors believe that there is no satisfactory marker for dialysis adequacy in AKI. Some authors reported that intermittent peritoneal dialysis was not adequate for treating AKI patients [24, 25]. Phu et al. showed that PD failed to keep optimal control of blood urea nitrogen (BUN) and creatinine levels compared with continuous venovenous hemodialysis, the latter having significantly lower mortality rate [24]. However, this study was frequently commented by others since their PD technique was not optimal: they produced PD solutions locally by using acetate buffer, used rigid peritoneal catheter, and performed manual PD exchanges with short procedure time leading to inadequate solute clearance and dialysis adequacy. The adequacy of PD in AKI was evaluated in a prospective, randomized, crossover trial that included 87 hypercatabolic patients [15]. This study showed that tidal PD and continuous equilibrated PD (CEPD), which is similar to but more intensive than continuous ambulatory peritoneal dialysis (CAPD), were adequate methods of maintaining BUN levels at about 65 mg/dL in mild and moderate hypercatabolic AKI patients in developing countries. Tidal PD provided better clearances at the same dialysis volume for a lower inpatient cost, and the only limitation was greater protein loss. In a prospective study, Gabriel et al. treated 30 AKI patients who received 236 dialysis sessions of PD with encouraging results for metabolic, electrolytic, and acid-base control [26]. They showed that high doses and PD using flexible catheter and cycler were an effective treatment of AKI providing high solute removal and sufficient dialysis dose with higher values than described in previous literature. An old but good method is the use of continuous flow PD (CFPD) [27]. This variant of PD utilizes two access points: one for inflow of dialysate and the other for outflow. Since there is no interruption of inflow to outflow, flow rates are determined only by the rate at which the draining catheter can efficiently drain the abdomen. With CFPD dialysate flow rates of up to 300 mL/min can be maintained through the peritoneum.

We believe that there are some important conclusions which can be derived on the basis of recent publications. First, the optimal treatment of AKI remains uncertain. Second, studies have shown the different therapeutic approaches to AKI. Third, in terms of PD, the optimal dose of dialysis is unclear. High-dose PD (weekly $Kt/V_{urea} > 3$) provides results comparable to those with HD. Whether lower doses in the range of 2.1, as suggested by some authors [28, 29], provide results comparable to those achieved with the higher doses remains to be determined, but data suggest that such a result may in fact be true. However, published studies have conflicting results (**Table 2**). In a recent review on PD dose in AKI [10], it was recommended that continuous forms of PD should be prescribed, with a minimum standardized $Kt/V_{urea}$ of at least 2.1 per week. Intermittent PD is the more commonly used modality in clinical practice with high level of uncertainty among professionals regarding the appropriate PD dose in AKI. This uncertainty is likely because of the paucity of strong evidence or consensus on this aspect. A systematic review of Chionh and coworkers showed that variable measures were used to represent dose and PD [29]. The total volume of peritoneal dialysate used was reported in eight studies as ranging from 13 to 70 L/d. Additional analysis of the relationship between PD dose and mortality was not possible.

| Reference | Std-$Kt/V_{urea}$ (per week) | $K_{urea}$ (mL/min) | $K_{Cr}$ (mL/min) | PD volume (L/d) |
|---|---|---|---|---|
| Ponce [27] | 3.5 ± 0.68 | NA | NA | 32.0–44.0 |
| Kilonzo et al. [7] | NA | NA | NA | 7.5 |
| Ponce et al. [30] | 3.6 | NA | NA | NA |
| George [29] | NA | 9.4 ± 4.9 | 10.5 ± 6.1 | NA |
| Gabriel et al. [2] | 3.6 ± 0.6 | 16.1 ± 4.0 | NA | 42.8 ± 5.72 |
| Gabriel [25] | 3.9 ± 0.6 | 17.3 ± 5.0 | 15.8 ± 4.2 | 43.2 ± 5.1 |
| Arogundade [31] | NA | NA | 8.1 ± 2.8 | 8.0 ± 0.6 |
| Phu [24] | NA | NA | NA | 70 |
| Chitalia et al. [15] | 1.8–2.4 | 10.6–19.8 | 5.8–6.8 | 13.0–26.3 |
| Thongboonkerd [32] | NA | 29.6 | 23.9 | 26.7 |
| Sonnenblick [33] | NA | NA | NA | 48.0 |

*Note*: Dose is represented by the standardized weekly $Kt/V_{urea}$ (std-$Kt/V_{urea}$), urea clearance ($K_{urea}$), creatinine clearance ($K_{Cr}$), and volume of PD effluent per day (PD volume). The dose is listed according to how the original article had presented the data: mean, mean ± SD, or range. PD, peritoneal dialysis; NA, results not available.

**Table 2.** Indicators of dose of PD.

In the absence of precise data, the clinician needs to exercise practical judgment in defining the optimal dose of PD. PD needs to be considered a reasonable treatment for AKI. The dose of PD that needs to be targeted for AKI remains uncertain and presents a challenge that is not different from the challenge presented in defining the optimal dose of HD or hemofiltration in the same situation. Clinical trials have not shown any advantage of increasing the dose of RRT above that obtained with alternate-day HD achieving a $Kt/V_{urea}$ of 1.2 per treatment.

Importantly, a $Kt/V_{urea}$ in that range can easily be reached with PD without the use of large volumes of solution. The authors emphasize the need to individualize therapy for each patient based on the clinical circumstances, severity of illness, hemodynamic stability, catabolic state, and so on [1, 10].

### 2.2. Types and methods of insertion of PD catheter

Peritoneal dialysis catheters could be divided in two groups, due to their placement and duration of use.

Acute peritoneal catheters have the same basic design: straight or slightly curved with holes at the distal end. These types of catheters are relatively rigid with an average diameter of 3 mm. By using wire or stylet, these catheters could be inserted, usually at the bedside. Also, these catheters are used immediately after the implantation procedure. They do not have cuffs and could be placed in the patient for three days. If longer use is anticipated, it is recommended that chronic catheter is to be inserted [34]. Because there are no protective cuffs, migration of bacteria from the skin to the subcutaneous tissue increases after three days. Since accidental dislodgments of acute catheter are quite common, care should be taken to provide proper catheter position once it is implanted [35].

Stylocath (Abbott Laboratories, North Chicago, IL) and the Trocath (Baxter Healthcare Corporation, Deerfield, IL) are the most used acute catheters with stylets. Guidewire an acute catheter designed to be inserted over a flexible catheter is available from Cook Co. (Bloomington, IN). The possibility of dialysis solution leak and high frequency of peritonitis are the main reasons why some centers prefer the use of the Tenckhoff catheter. Tenckhoff recommended the use of a single-cuff catheter for acute cases [36].

Chronic peritoneal catheters are usually constructed from silicone rubber or polyurethane. Adult catheters have outer diameter of 5 mm and three internal diameters: 2.16, 3.1, and 3.5 mm. They have two cuffs as a protection from infections. These cuffs will provoke local inflammatory response after formation of scar tissue. As a result, this tissue will be an anchor for catheter. The catheter should function for several years [37]. Peritonitis could be treated without removal of these catheters [38].

In resource-poor settings, some improvised devices could be used: nasogastric tube, rubber catheter, and intercostal drainage catheter. All of these devices must be inserted surgically and are more prone to different complications due to their design [10]. Intraperitoneal part of PD catheters has four basic designs: straight Tenckhoff with side holes on distal end, coiled Tenckhoff with coiled portion with side holes, straight Tenckhoff with perpendicular silicone disc also known as an Oreopoulos-Zellerman or Toronto Western Hospital catheter, and T-shaped catheter with grooved limbs that position against the peritoneum.

Latest guidelines recommend the use of flexible peritoneal catheters for acute PD in cases where resources and expertise exist [39]. Otherwise, rigid stylet catheters or improvised catheters could be used as a lifesaving device. Wong et al. compared flexible Tenckhoff catheters and rigid stylet catheters in children who underwent acute PD. They found fewer complications with flexible catheters and significantly longer catheter survival [40]. Good function of catheter demands several specifications: the tip should be placed in the pelvic cavity; catheter is implanted in the paramedian lower abdomen. Several methods of placement are used. Percutaneous non-visualized method is a blind method, and fluoroscopy could be used. Methods with direct visualization are surgical minilaparotomy, peritoneoscopy, or open surgical dissection. Some procedures could be done as a bedside procedure. Catheters should be tunneled in order to reduce peritonitis and peri-catheter leaks [10] **(Table 3)**.

| Type | Advantage | Disadvantage |
|---|---|---|
| Rigid stylet catheter | Cheap | More dysfunctions |
| | Bedside procedure | Flow-related problems |
| | Easily removed | Risk of abdominal organ injury |
| Flexible | Better flow | Expensive |
| | Less chance for organ perforation, less infection and leaks | Necessary training prior to implantation<br>Easily migrated |
| | Bedside procedure | |
| Improvised devices | Inexpensive | Infections, leaks, flow-related problem |
| | Easily available | Difficult to connect |

**Table 3.** Main characteristics of flexible, rigid, and improvised devices for acute PD.

No method of insertion is superior overall to the others [41]. Choice of method will depend on patient conditions and skills and expertise of medical staff. It is worth to mention that ISPD recommends that "insertion by nephrologists is safe and functional results equate to those inserted surgically." Also, the same guideline recommends "that nephrologists receive training and be permitted to insert these catheters to ensure timely dialysis in the emergency setting." In their survey, Sampathkumar et al. show that with a skilled nephrologist subcutaneous placement could be used very effectively to provide fast dialysis approach [42]. Similar results were found in several studies elsewhere [43].

Kumar et al. described a case from a large-scale disaster in which human life was saved by a relatively inexperienced doctor who had basic skills in catheter insertion [8].

The most common used methods for insertion of PD catheter are surgical, laparoscopic, peritoneoscopic, and blind techniques (**Table 4**). In 1968, Tenckhoff and Schechter were the first to describe a percutaneous non-visualized method of catheter placement. Brewer in 1972 invented open placement as a mini-surgical laparotomy. Since that, several new approaches were described, namely, laparoscopic as the newest one. Blind techniques include the Seldinger technique, the trochar method, and the fluoroscopic guidance.

| Name | Advantage | Disadvantage |
|---|---|---|
| Percutaneous | Bedside | Risk of abdominal injury |
| | Minimal skill | Not suitable for patients with previous interventions |
| Open surgical | Available in most hospitals | Surgical scheduling |
| | Relatively cheap compared to laparoscopic | |
| Laparoscopy | Ability to reach pelvis under vision | Skilled personnel |
| | Low leak | Expensive |
| | Additional procedures possible | |

**Table 4.** Different implantation techniques of PD catheter.

Prior to implantation, the patient is advised to empty the bladder, and antibiotics are administered. Adequate procedure will eliminate surgical complication and reduce risk for transfer to HD. The most important determinants of catheter outcome are placement technique and skill of operator. There are strong recommendations from several international scientific bodies that antibiotics should be used prior to implantation of catheter.

Protocols for antibiotic prophylaxis prior to catheter insertion should be guided by the local infectious disease guidelines. The UK Renal Association and ERA-EDTA stated that antibiotics should and must be used. ISPD in its 2010 guidelines recommends that "renal units should have clear protocols for perioperative catheter care, including the use of antibiotic prophylaxis" [44]. The usual approach is single-dose intravenous route prior to insertion. Gadallah and colleagues in their research included several groups of patients who were given cefazolin and vancomycin and a control group without any drugs. The vancomycin group had the least infectious complications, and the protocol they recommended was 1 g vancomycin i.v. single dose 12 h before peritoneal catheter placement procedures. This dosage was superior to cefazolin in preventing possible early infection due to catheter placement [45]. Later, Strippoli et al. conducted meta-analysis which included four studies with 335 patients in total. They concluded that perioperative antibiotic prophylaxis reduced infection significantly compared to nonantibiotic group. There was no significant difference in the risk of exit site/tunnel infection [46]. Based on mentioned research, ISPD guidelines recommend that vancomycin should be part in any protocol according to potential risk and benefits of patient [47].

### 2.3. Indications and contraindications of acute PD

The indications for acute PD can be divided into two groups: renal and nonrenal (**Table 5**).

| Indications of acute PD | | PD is contraindicated in the following clinical situations |
|---|---|---|
| **Renal indications** | **Nonrenal indications** | |
| RRT in the treatment of AKI in children<br>Hemodynamically unstable patients<br>The presence of bleeding diathesis or hemorrhagic conditions contra indicating placement of vascular access for hemodialysis or anti coagulation<br>Patients with difficult vascular access placement<br>Removal of high-molecular weight toxins (10 kDa) | Acute pancreatitis<br>Clinically significant hypothermia or hyperthermia<br>Refractory heart failure<br>Liver failure<br>Infusion of drugs and nutrients as a supportive therapy in critically ill patients | Recent abdominal surgery<br>Pleuroperitoneal communication<br>Diaphragmatic severe respiratory failure<br>Life-threatening hyperkalemia not responding to medical therapy<br>Extremely hypercatabolic state<br>Severe volume overload in a patient not on a ventilator<br>Severe gastroesophageal reflux disease<br>Low peritoneal clearance<br>Fecal or fungal peritonitis<br>Abdominal wall cellulitis<br>AKI in pregnancy |

**Table 5.** Renal and nonrenal indications and contraindications of PD in AKI.

### 2.3.1. *Renal indications*

Peritoneal dialysis is an advantageous modality for RRT in AKI (**Table 5**). In many of the studies of PD versus HD for AKI, the reason for improved survival in the PD group was related to an increased rate of renal recovery. It is already known that in patients with ESRD, treatment by PD resulted in better preservation of intrinsic renal function than treatment by intermittent HD. This preservation of renal function is important because it maintains endocrine function of the kidneys, diminishes the clearance requirements for dialysis, and minimizes ultrafiltration and physiologic stress during dialysis. On the other hand, hemodialysis has several known nephrotoxic effects such as generation of inflammatory mediators by extracorporeal circuit, rapid decrease in osmolality, and vascular volume, diminishing renal perfusion. All of the above may influence renal recovery during the course of AKI. PD can easily meet treatment goals for AKI patients, maintaining adequate fluid, electrolyte, and acid base balances. It also allows the use of other supportive measures without limitation until the recovery of renal function. However, as compared to HD, PD is less effective in severe acute illnesses like pulmonary edema, poisoning, or drug overdose, and hypercatabolic states. Several reports suggest that patients with AKI secondary to atheroembolic renal disease may have a better chance of recovery if PD is used over HD [48]. It has also been reported that PD has a beneficial role in recovery of renal function in patients with renal failure due to malignant hypertension [49]. In resource-poor countries, the cost, practicability, and feasibility of CRRT may be limiting factors, whereas peritoneal dialysis is relatively simple and inexpensive and is more widely used. Simplicity of PD permits interns and postgraduate students to be trained to manage AKI earlier at primary care centers, thus avoiding the delay caused by referring critically ill patients to nephrologist or ICU. Finally, even in developed countries, a major catastrophe can cause severe damage to the infrastructure. PD is an alternative when reliable power, clean water supply, and facilities for water treatment are unavailable.

Small molecular clearance is lower with PD than that achieved with conventional HD due to characteristics of peritoneal dialysate. However, the clearance of higher molecular weight solutes is higher with continuous PD than with HD. Ultrafiltration rate gradually decreases during PD due to continuous fall of glucose in dialysate fluid [30].

#### 2.3.1.1. *Nonrenal indications for acute PD*

PD can be used in various extrarenal conditions (**Table 2**). In acute hemorrhagic pancreatitis, hypothermia or hyperthermia, and congestive heart failure, PD could be used if patient does not respond to conventional therapy [39, 50]. In patients with fulminant liver failure, PD has been used because it avoids the need for anticoagulation [51]. Finally, PD may help in the removal of toxins like ammonia, bilirubin, and free fatty acids. On the other hand, PD may be used as route for delivery of nutrients like glucose and amino acids and certain drugs in severely ill patients admitted to intensive care unit [52].

#### 2.3.1.2. *Contraindications to acute PD*

There are several relative contraindications to acute PD (**Table 3**): recent operation with abdominal drainage, peritonitis (fecal or fungal), and known pleuroperitoneal fistula (after cardiothoracic surgery). The presence of abdominal hernia or intra-abdominal adhesions might make PD difficult. PD may be relatively contraindicated in the presence of abdominal wall cellulitis or severe gastroesophageal reflux disease, adynamic ileus, and recent aortic graft (<6 months). PD is noneffective in treatment of life-threatening hyperkalemia. The use of PD in hyperkalemia should be employed in situations when HD is not available. Also, PD is not the best treatment modality in patients with a high load of azotemia [53].

### 2.4. Limitations of PD in AKI

Though easy and reliable, PD has some limitations in the treatment of AKI [54], and one of them and the most important is less efficacy for severe acute pulmonary edema and in life-threatening hyperkalemia as well as being its need for an intact peritoneal cavity with adequate peritoneal clearance capacity. Unlike HD, ultrafiltration and clearance cannot be exactly predicted in PD patients. The major criticism of PD is the low clearance of uremic toxins; the clearance of low-molecular weight toxins is lower than for other therapies (continuous arteriovenous hemofiltration, continuous venovenous hemofiltration, and daily HD). It is apparent that PD with a modest dialysate use of 1 L/h is less efficient than other modalities for urea and creatinine but is similarly efficient in removal of larger molecules such as vitamin B12. It is likely that larger-molecular weight toxins are the real cause of uremic illness, and PD is quite effective in removing various anionic organic compounds that function as middle molecules. Small molecular clearance may be increased by increasing flow rate of dialysate to 1.5–1.0 L/h or more. Tidal peritoneal dialysis can easily deliver 2 L/h into and out of the peritoneum. Infectious, mechanical, and metabolic complications may be major problems. The incidence of peritonitis in PD therapy of AKI is much different than in PD therapy. Previous studies have reported a 12–25% incidence of peritonitis. If peritonitis is detected during therapy of AKI, it usually occurs within 2 or 3 days of starting therapy [39]. This indicates that PD may detect contamination of the peritoneum that predates the implementation of PD. There is predominance of *Staphylococcus epidermidis* and *Candida* (in debilitated patients undergoing antibiotic therapies) but also mixed infections [55]. Peritonitis during PD therapy does not result in septicemia in AKI patients. This is a much different outcome than catheter-related infections during hemodialysis or continuous therapies which frequently result in septicemia. The increasing use of automated PD via flexible catheter has led to a reduction in peritonitis frequency. Studies have shown that mechanical complications occur in fewer than 10% of patients due to immediate use just after catheter insertion [26]. Also, there is controversy about abdominal distension leading to reduced diaphragm mobilization and consequently about pulmonary compliance. Protein losses may play an important role, mainly during peritonitis. It may exacerbate conditions in undernourished, critically ill patients with AKI. It was measured that total weekly protein losses were around 45 g in intermittent and 62 g in continuous peritoneal dialysis (CPD); albumin accounted for approximately half of this loss. Despite this depletion, plasma albumin and total protein levels were not decreased [56]. However, large variability among individuals was seen, and peritonitis was the only factor influencing these losses. This observation was reported by Gabriel et al. who reported no significant difference between median plasma albumin values obtained before and after CPD session (median 2.6 g/dL) despite considerable losses in protein (median 21.7 g/day). The authors concluded that dialysate protein loss, although significant, was not a limiting factor for using CPD. In these situations, it is necessary to increase patient's protein ingestion which should be 1.5 g/kg/day. The fact that PD results in protein loss is generally considered a nutritional problem. However, this loss may contribute to the chemical effectiveness of the PD. In patients with hemolytic uremic syndrome, PD significantly reduces plasminogen activator inhibitor type 1 (PAI-1) which inhibits fibrinolysis in hemolytic uremic syndrome [57]. Most of the organic anions removed by PD in uremic patients are in fact strongly bound to protein, so protein loss increases their clearance. These protein-bound organic anions act as middle molecules, and the presence of protein within the dialysate facilitates the transfer of these compounds into the peritoneum. The peritoneal transfer of proteins can be increased by application of hypertonic solutions; the globulin removal by PD on a daily basis could equal or exceed daily therapeutic plasmapheresis [58]. Hyperglycemia is another metabolic complication resulting from PD with glucose-based solutions. Therefore, it is necessary to closely monitor glucose metabolism even by using insulin via continuous infusion pump [15]. When comparing the overall risk of each type of therapy for AKI, there are marked differences between continuous venovenous hemofiltration, continuous venovenous hemodialysis, HD, and PD. The blood treatment therapies have a significant risk of septicemia, low flow from blood access, hypotension, membrane clothing, and bleeding. PD therapy includes risk of PD catheter outflow failure, hyperglycemia, and asymptomatic peritonitis. There are controversies about the influence of PD on respiratory system in critically ill patients. In ICU settings where patients are on ventilation, PD using high volume may impair diaphragmatic movement, and this should be taken into consideration while profiling the patient. As a result, pulmonary compliance and ventilation are impaired. Venous return is also reduced leading to hypotension and consequently to organ and tissue hypoperfusion which favor acidosis. The effective peritoneal blood flow in uremic patients during dialysis is 100 mL/min [39] and cannot be increased as in the case of CRRT and HD. Leblanc et al. [59] showed that although it reduces pulmonary volume, characteristics of vital capacity and expiratory volume remain unaltered. They concluded that PD is rarely associated with ventilatory impairment in patients without pulmonary pathologies. However, it must be emphasized that in nearly all the abovementioned situations, PD may be tried as the initial RRT modality and prescription adjusted to get optimum dialysis and ultrafiltration.

### 2.5. Prescription of PD in AKI

After the insertion of an acute or chronic peritoneal catheter (preferably chronic if possible), PD orders need to be individualized depending upon the hemodynamic status of the patient, laboratory work, and volume status. The components of PD orders are multiple and involve the following: length of the dialysis session, dialysate composition, exchange volume, inflow and outflow periods, dwell time, number of exchanges, additives, and monitoring of fluid balance.

The length of a PD session can vary depending on the cause and duration of AKI, the need for water and solute removal, and the risk of infection although usual dialysis session lasts for 48–72 h, and each exchange is done over 1 h. PD fluid is available in different glucose concentrations and various electrolyte concentrations (**Table 6**). It should be warmed to body temperature prior to infusion to avoid enhanced solute transport.

| Type | $Na^+$ | $K^+$ | $Ca^{2+}$ | $Mg^{2+}$ | $Cl^-$ | $HCO_3^-$ | Lactate | pH | Osm. |
|---|---|---|---|---|---|---|---|---|---|
| Stay safe 1.5% | 132 | | 2.5 | 0.5 | 95 | | 40 | 5.5 | 344 |
| Dianeal 1.5% | 132 | | 2.5 | 0.25 | 95 | | 35 | 5.2 | 344 |

*Note*: Na = sodium; K = potassium; Ca = calcium; Mg = magnesium; Cl = chlorine; $HCO_3$ = bicarbonate; osm. = osmolarity

**Table 6.** Typical composition of commercially available PD fluid.

| Glucose (g/dL) | Fluid osmolarity (mOsm/L) | Ultrafiltrate volume (mL per exchange over 1 h) |
|---|---|---|
| 1.5 | 346 | 50–150 |
| 2.5 | 396 | 100–300 |
| 4.25 | 485 | 300–400 |

**Table 7.** Dialysis fluid glucose concentration.

To obtain better ultrafiltration, it is reasonable to initiate acute PD in most patients with the 2.5 g/dL PD fluid. Using standard regimen, different amounts of fluid can be removed over a

24-h period: 2.5 L with 1.5 g/dL glucose, 4.5 L with 2.5 g/dL glucose, and 8.5 L with 4.25 g/dL glucose. Various types of glucose concentration are available to be used in acute PD prescription (**Tables 6** and **7**).

(1) 1.5 g/dL PD fluid contains 27.2 g of glucose in 2 L bag (ultrafiltration of 50–150 mL/h / 2 L, 60 min exchange time). It is the most commonly used fluid in acute PD; (2) 2.5 g/dL PD fluid contains 45.4 g of glucose in 2 L bag (ultrafiltration of 100–300 mL/h/2 L, 60 min exchange time); (3) 4.25 g/dL PD fluid contains 77.2 g of glucose in 2 L bag (ultrafiltration of 300–400 mL/h/2 L, 60 min exchange time). This hypertonic fluid is usually used in patients with volume overload like congestive heart failure. But its longer use can induce hemodynamic instability due to massive ultrafiltration. Usually, this degree of UF is not required and can use combination of glucose concentrations to attain level of UF desired.

PD orders need to be individualized depending upon hemodynamic status of the patient and volume status. After confirmation that PD catheter is adequately inserted and has no problems with flow of the fluid [35], PD orders need to be reviewed and written daily (**Table 8**).

| Nursing orders | Renal physician to be notified immediately for the following situations |
|---|---|
| Dialysis session length … hours | Poor dialysate flow |
| Dialysis volume per exchange … L | Severe abdominal pain or distention |
| Dialysis dextrose concentration, % | Change in color of dialysate, bloody, or cloudy drainage |
| Inflow time … min dwell time; outflow time… | Dialysate leak or purulent drainage around catheter exit site |
| Vital signs q … hours | Blood pressure of … mm Hg |
| Weigh patient q … hours | Respiratory rate of ≥ … per minute or severe shortness of breath in non-ventilated patient |
| Warm dialysate fluid to body temperature | Temperature of ≥ … C |
| Maintain strict intake and output | Two consecutive positive exchanges |
| Additives to dialysate: heparin, yes/no; insulin, yes/no; potassium, yes/no | Single-positive exchange balance if negative balance exceeds … L over … hours |
| Vancomycin … mg/L of exchange, other … mg/L of exchange; other antibiotic … mg/L | Notification of abnormal laboratory values |
| Catheter care and dressing change everyday | |
| Full chemistry panel including blood glucose level to be done every 12 h each day during dialysis | |
| 15 ml of dialysate fluid from catheter every morning during dialysis and send it for cell count with differential, gram staining, and culture; yes/no | |

**Table 8.** Acute PD orders.

The most practical way to achieve fluid removal is by mixing and matching low- and high-glucose concentration adequate fluid. Exchange volume is the amount of PD fluid instilled into the peritoneal cavity during an exchange. The volume instilled depends on the intraperitoneal pressure (IPP), the presence of pulmonary disease or mechanical ventilation, and the presence of abdominal hernia. An average-sized adult can tolerate 2 L exchanges, but in smaller patients, those with pulmonary disease or those with abdominal or inguinal hernias, the exchange volume should be reduced.

The intraperitoneal pressure rises linearly with higher volume of intraperitoneal fluid used. Intraperitoneal pressure is higher in patients with higher body mass index. Age, gender, weight, height, body surface area, and diabetes mellitus do not correlate with IPP [60]. Low-PDF volume is used after the PD catheter placement to avoid leakage. The volume is gradually increased over the next three or four days as tolerated by the patient. Inflow time is the time required to instill the PD fluid into the peritoneal cavity under the effect of gravity. The time is usually 10–15 min. It should be kept to minimal to maximize efficiency of peritoneal dialysis.

Dwell time is the time period for which the exchange volume stays in the intraperitoneal cavity which is usually 30 min in the single acute peritoneal dialysis exchange. A dwell time of less than 30 min is usually not adequate [61]. The dwell time for patients on acute CPD is about 3–6 h which can be shortened to increase the total number of exchanges to improve solute clearance.

Outflow time is the time required to drain effluent dialysate after dwell which takes place under the effect of gravity. It is usually takes 20–30 min to complete [62]. If incomplete, drainage can cause a rise in intra-abdominal pressure causing respiratory embarrassment or abdominal discomfort. The usual number of exchanges is about 24/day with standard acute PD and approximately 4–6/day with CPD.

Some drugs can be added to the PD fluid to treat certain specific conditions. Some of these drugs are the following:

*Potassium.* Normally, there is no potassium in the dialysis fluid, but potassium can be added to the PD fluid in hypokalemic patients. Usually 3–4 mmol/L is added to maintain normokalemia [10].

*Insulin.* Usually insulin is used in diabetic patients on PD for glycemic control. Intraperitoneal insulin is usually added to the PD fluid, and the dose is adjusted based on frequent blood glucose monitoring. It should be avoided in last 2–3 exchanges to prevent postdialysis hypoglycemia.

As glucose concentration rises, an increasing insulin dose in the dialysis bag is needed as follows: 4–5 units/L for 1.5 g/dL PD fluid, 5–7 units/L for 2.5 g/dL PD fluid, and 7–10 units/L for 4.25 g/dL PD fluid.

*Anticoagulants.* Heparin is used to prevent clot formation. Usually a dose of 500 units/L is given after plugs, or strands of fibrin are visible on the drained fluid [10]. There is no systemic absorption of heparin through peritoneum and there is no systemic anticoagulation risk when heparin is used intraperitoneally.

*Antibiotics.* Intraperitoneal administration of antibiotics is efficient with a huge variety of antibiotics which can be administered intraperitoneally. This route is preferred to intravenous dosing for treating peritonitis. Both intermittent and dosing of antibiotics are equally efficacious. Empiric treatment of peritonitis should start immediately and should have both gram-positive and gram-negative coverage. Results of culture and sensitivity should be followed, and antibiotics should be changed based on sensitivity of the organism. Most patients show considerable clinical improvement within 48 h of initiation of antibiotic treatment. The reader should refer to the International Society of Peritoneal Dialysis guidelines regarding doses of various antibiotics used intraperitoneally in PD for treatment of peritonitis [10, 63].

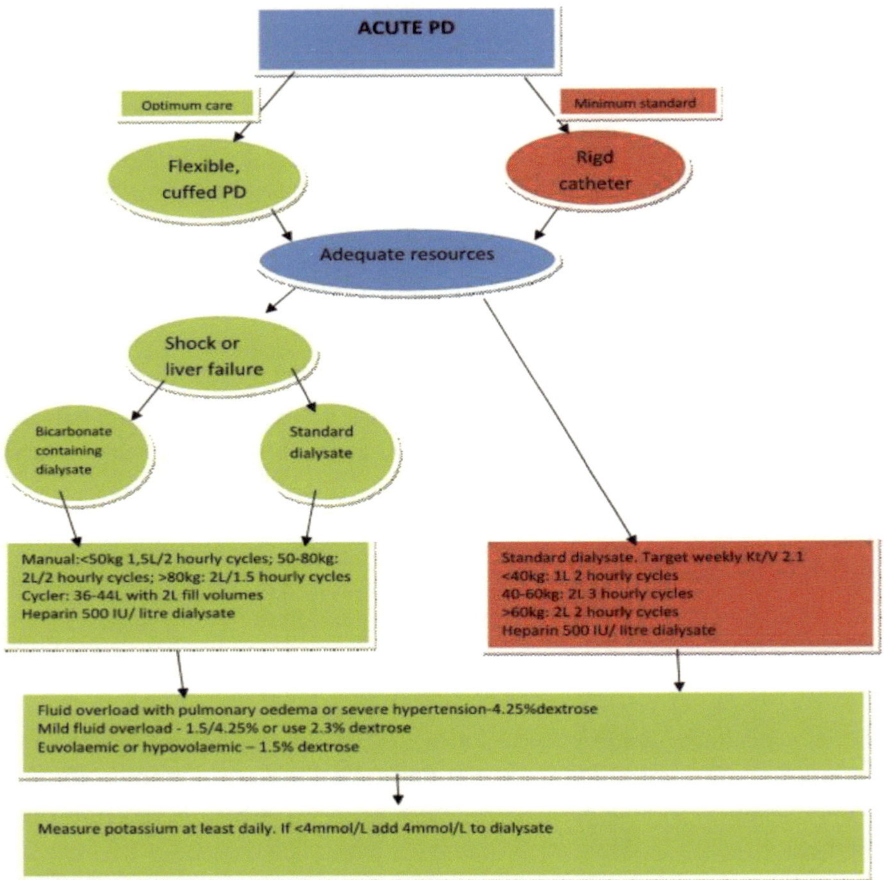


**Figure 1.** The proposed dosing algorithm for PD in AKI.

## 2.6. ISPD guidelines for PD in AKI

ISPD guidelines [10] state that PD should be considered as a suitable method for RRT in AKI. Flexible peritoneal catheters should be preferred. Catheter insertion by a nephrologist is safe and functional results equal that of surgical insertion. Preoperative prophylactic antibiotics such as first-generation cephalosporins or vancomycin reduce the incidence of peritonitis among PD patients [46]. ISPD recommends the use of PD fluids with bicarbonate as the buffer in patients with shock or liver failure. Fluid overload is to be avoided, and ultrafiltration can be increased by raising the concentration of dextrose and shortening the cycle duration (**Figure 1**).

### 2.7. Complications of PD for AKI

There are a number of potential complications associated with the use of acute PD.

Peritonitis is the most common complication in PD, in AKI, as well as in chronic kidney disease (CKD), so the treatment of peritonitis is different: due to more rapid exchanges generally performed with acute PD than chronic PD, antibiotics should be given intraperitoneally and with every exchange.

Another important complication is mechanical or catheter-related problems. Mechanical complications are abdominal pain, discomfort, intra-abdominal hemorrhage, bowel perforation, catheter malfunction, and peritoneal fluid leakage. Perforation of abdominal organs, namely, bladder, is a rare complication. It is made by using the blind methods. Frequency of perforation reported in previous percutaneous studies is very low (around 1%) [43].

In their study, Mittal and all reported of 2% bleeding complication mainly connected with anticoagulation therapy. So, they recommended withdrawal of this drug at least 24 h prior to intervention [64].

Catheter obstruction may be a result of fibrin blockage of the catheter or tubing or displacement ± omental wrapping of the catheter. Leakage of peritoneal fluid is most often seen in the older patients and also in those who are obese and with previous abdominal operation. Other factors that can contribute to peritoneal fluid leakage are diabetes mellitus, steroid use, and multiparity.

Pulmonal complications in acute PD could be atelectasis, pneumonia, aspiration, and pleural effusion. All these complications are due to increased intra-abdominal pressure. Rinsing the catheter with sterile saline using sterile technique may remove the blockage. Once flow is reestablished, 1,000 units of heparin will be added to each liter of PD fluid. Methods for manipulating displaced PD catheters could include the use of guidewire manipulation and laxatives. If these methods fail, the catheter should be replaced using the original catheter way into the peritoneum. Loss of protein from the peritoneum in patients on chronic PD varies in different studies from 6.2 to 12.8 g/day or even 48 g during episodes of peritonitis.

Care should be taken to ensure that adequate protein intake occurs aiming for approximately 1.2 g/kg of protein per day. Protein loss is in association with increased mortality in those patients with a negative protein balance.

Due to the high glucose concentration in PD fluid, there is a tendency to hyperglycemia in acute PD which decreases osmotic gradient. It should be treated to enable optimal ultrafiltration. In diabetic patients who are treated with insulin in peritoneal solution, hypoglycemia could occur. Acid-base imbalance could be the result of simultaneous therapy with bicarbonate with the aim of fast correction of metabolic acidosis. On the other hand, hypernatremia is the result of high ultrafiltration rate due to hyperosmotic solutions. Hypokalemia is the result of using solutions without potassium [10].

| Study (authors) | Type | Country | Period | ICU pts (%) | Causes of AKI | *N* | Mortality (%) |
|---|---|---|---|---|---|---|---|
| Ponce et al. [30] | Pros. | Brazil | 2004/2014 | 66.8 | Sepsis (53.2%), ATN (26.9%), others (19.9%) | 301 | 59.8 |
| Ponce [27] | Pros. | Brazil | 2004/2011 | NA | Sepsis (41.1%), ATN (34.1%) | 150 | 57.3 |
| Kilonzo et al. [7] | Retr. | Tanzania | 2009/2011 | NA | ATN (40.0%), GN (20.0%) | 14 | 21.4 |
| Ponce [30] | Pros. | Brazil | 2005/2007 | NA | Sepsis (49.5%), heart failure (23.5%), postsurgery (12.5%) | 61 | 54.1 |
| Hayat et al. [66] | Retr. | India | 2004/2005 | NA | Gastroenteritis (75.0%) | 43 | 10.0 |
| Gabriel et al. [26] | Pros. | Brazil | 2004 | 76.0 | Ischemic (67%), mixed (33%) | 30 | 57.0 |
| Chitalia et al. [15] | Pros. | India | NA | NA | Prerenal (30.0%), leptospirosis (17.2%), others (13.8%) | 87 | 1.1 |
| Thongboonkerd [32] | Pros. | Thailand | NA | 100.0 | Shock (50%), nonshock (50%) | 20 | 15.0 |
| Howdieshell et al. [67] | Retr. | USA | 1989/1990 | 100.0 | Trauma-related (100%) | 5 | 40.0 |
| Sonnenblick [33] | Retr. | Israel | 1975/1986 | 100.0 | Sepsis (38.6%), prerenal (36.4%), others (25%) | 44 | 70.5 |
| Ojogwu [68] | Pros. | Nigeria | NA | NA | Hypertensive crisis (100%) | 20 | 100 |
| Cameron et al. [69] | Retr. | UK | 1965/1967 | NA | Postcardiac (33.3%) and postaortic surgery (33.3%) | 9 | 66.7 |

**Table 9.** AKI patients treated with PD only.

## 2.8. PD and renal outcome in patients with AKI

In many of the studies of PD versus HD for AKI [10, 61], the reason for improved survival in the PD group was related to an increased rate of renal recovery (**Tables 9** and **10**). It is already known that in patients with end stage renal disease (ESRD), treatment by CAPD resulted in better preservation of intrinsic renal function than treatment by intermittent HD. This preservation of renal function is important because it maintains endocrine function of the kidneys, diminishes the clearance requirements for dialysis, and minimizes ultrafiltration and physiologic stress during dialysis. On the other hand, hemodialysis has several known nephrotoxic effects such as generation of inflammatory mediators by extracorporeal circuit and rapid decrease in osmolality and vascular volume, diminishing renal perfusion. All of the above may influence renal recovery during the course of AKI. By contrast, CAPD may help to maintain renal perfusion by smaller daily variation in body weight, more constant blood pressure and continuous mild overhydration, persistent high blood osmolality, and continuous removal of proteins from the blood including $\beta_2$-micoglobulin, albumin, plasminogen activator inhibitor type 1 (PAI-1), and immunoglobulins [65]. These some physiologic and chemical benefits may account for the highest recovery of renal function in most studies, in patients with AKI treated by PD than HD.

The characteristics of the relevant studies are summarized in **Tables 9** and **10**. The number of patients, results, and percentages represents only patients who had RRT. Thirteen studies were descriptive in nature, in which PD was the only mode of RRT including 597 patients. Three studies (Ponce, Thongboonkerd) compared different subtypes of PD. In 11 studies, there was a comparing group treated with EBP (**Table 9**): seven studies were cohort studies, whereas four studies were prospective randomized clinical trials (RCTs). One study (Chow YW) described two distinct cohorts of patients in 1994 and 2004, and the data from each cohort were analyzed separately. In one RCT (Arogundade), only 8 of 40 patients had AKI; only these patients were included in the analysis. Details of the PD technique were often not reported. Where data were available, the studies used either rigid catheters or flexible Tenckhoff catheters. The automated cycler was used in four studies, and closed drainage systems were commonly used. As buffer, lactate (10 studies), acetate (3), and bicarbonate (1) were used. The majority (19 of 24) of these studies came from low-resource regions, such as Asia, Africa, and South America. From the developed countries such as Canada, the United States, the United Kingdom, and Australia, there was only one study research. Over one-half of the studies were published in the year 2000 or later; six studies were published before 1990. The last study by Ponce et al. has been published from 2004 to 2014 [30, 75]. The predominant cause of AKI is sepsis, and mortality is 59.8%. In the studies that used PD only, fourteen studies were analyzed, and from this number, five studies have been conducted predominantly in the ICU setting. The mortality was 39.3%, whereas reported mortality in the individual studies ranged from 1.1 to 100%. However, in the studies that used PD or EBP, four studies have been conducted only in the ICU, and studies were RCTs. In the present studies, 392 patients underwent PD, whereas 567 patients underwent EBP. For PD patients, mortality rate is ranged from 25 to 75.8%, except for two studies with 0% mortality. On the other hand, mortality for EBP patients ranged from 15 to 84% in individual studies. The total mortality was 58% for PD and 56.1% for EBP. Chionh and colleagues [29] have found among the observational studies that there was no significant difference in mortality between PD and EBP (odds ratio, 0.9 confidence interval, 0.53–1.71).

Finally, on the basis of this research, we could have several important findings. There is an evident lack of good-quality data, and studies showed no difference in mortality between PD and EBP. PD dose and some important outcomes (renal recovery, PD-related complications) were underreported.

| Study (authors) | Type | Country | Period | ICU pts (%) | EBP used | Causes of AKI | PD | EBP | Overall mort. (%) |
|---|---|---|---|---|---|---|---|---|---|
| | | | | | | | Mort. (%) | Mort. (%) | |
| Watcharotone et al. [11] | Retr. | Thailand | 2005/2009 | 69.7 | Int. HD | NA | 75.8 | 62.7 | 68.3 |
| George [29] | RCT | India | 2005/2008 | 100 | CVVHDF | Sepsis (38%), prerenal (34%), leptospirosis (10%), snake bite (6%) | 72 | 84 | 78 |
| Gabriel et al. [3] | RCT | Brazil | 2004/2006 | 77.4 | Daily HD | Sepsis (44.5%), prerenal (39.2%), postsurgery (22.5%) | 58 | 53 | 55.5 |
| Chow et al. [70] | Pros. | Malaysia | 2004/2005 | 13.3 | Int. HD, CVVHDF | Prerenal (53.5%), sepsis (37.9%), toxins (6.2%) | 12 | 75 | 46.7 |
| Mahajan et al. [71] | Retr. | India | 2000/2004 | NA | Int. HD | Prerenal (33%), sepsis (21.6%), toxins (16.1%) | 46 | 67.6 | 53.8 |
| Arogundade [31] | RCT | Nigeria | 1998/2001 | NA | Int. HD | Sepsis (87.5%), obstruction (12.5%) | 0 | 0 | 0 |
| Chow et al. [70] | Pros. | Malaysia | 1994 | 29.5 | Int. HD, CVVHDF | Prerenal (43.6%), sepsis (41%), toxins (10.3%) | 66.7 | 66.7 | 66.7 |
| Phu [24] | RCT | Vietnam | 1993/1998 | 100 | CVVHDF | Malaria (68.6%), sepsis (31.4%) | 17 | 15% | 31.5 |
| Kumar et al. [8] | Retr. | India | 1987/1998 | NA | Int. HD | Diarrheal illness (100%) | 25 | 66.7 | 60 |
| Bellomo et al. [72] | Retr. | Australia | 1983/1993 | 100 | HDF, Int. HD | Sepsis (66%) | 12 | 63.8 | 64.5 |
| Hadidy et al. [73] | Retr. | Syria | 1980/2006 | NA | Int. HD | Obstruction, surgery, trauma 64%; pregnancy | 0 | 33.8 | 30.9 |
| Werb and Linton [74] | Retr. | Canada | 1974/2006 | 100 | Int. HD | Sepsis (28%), prerenal (17%) | 69.2 | 65 | 65.5 |

**Table 10.** AKI patients treated with either PD or extracorporeal blood purification.

Possible confounders are identified in this chapter. Time span and different epidemiologies of AKI were most visible. The studies last over four decades in which approach and technical issues evolve significantly. HD was changed from imprecise machines with low efficiency and flux bioincompatible membranes that were with those dialyzers with high efficiency and high flux for EBP. PD evolved from manual exchanges at low doses to automated PD and higher doses. We now tend to see older patients with multiple comorbid conditions who have undergone interventions, such as radiocontrast procedures, high-risk surgery, and invasive ICU care [29]. Also, selection bias is likely among the nonrandomized studies. Physician's personal opinion and experience on different treatment modalities are the main base for patient's selection in studies.

## 3. Conclusions

Adequate treatment for most AKI patients without contraindications for PD use is based on careful prescription and accurate measurement of efficiency, which allows adequate metabolic and fluid control. Age and sepsis were risk factors associated with death, whereas follow-up time, urine output, UF, and nitrogen balance were protective factors against mortality.

Recently, interest in using PD to manage AKI patients has been increasing. It is frequently used in developing countries because of its advantages for this surrounding. However, in those countries, the infrastructure for quality research is often lacking. There is lack of evidence on important information for standardized treatment such as indications, dosing, volumes, technical failure, and mortality. But, so far, results have shown that critically ill patients can be successfully treated by PD.

PD is an acceptable form of treatment in patients with AKI. Recent studies have suggested that outcomes with PD are as good as with extracorporeal RRTs. While the ISPD guidelines as well as the recently published "Update on PD" [76] focus on optimal treatment algorithms, it is important to keep in mind that treatment patterns need to be developed in accordance with individual patient needs. In low-resource settings, flexibility and appropriate adjustments in treatment patterns may need to be made. According our national renal patient registry, PD was only 2.6% in 2015 to treat ESRD patients only. We have very little experience in using PD for AKI. Our center had been using AIPD even though rarely. We hope this chapter will encourage the application of this method not only in chronic kidney disease but also in AKI.

Looking globally, the majority of the world population lives in developing countries with two-thirds or below the poverty line. AKI is common in such populations due to a variety of causes. Dialysis modality should be available to save lives. Based on available information, we may conclude that PD is as suitable as EBP to treat AKI.

PD may be a viable option for treatment because there is no significant difference in outcomes between PD and EBP. In the absence of precise data, the clinician needs to exercise judgment in selecting a dialysis modality. The choice should depend on the clinical status of the patient as well as the expertise and resources of the center. Well-designed and powered randomized trials are needed to evaluate clinically important outcomes as well as cost. Standardized reporting of technique, dose, complications, and cost like the Utstein style should be encouraged for observational studies.

## Author details

Damir Rebić* and Vedad Herenda

*Address all correspondence to: damir.rebic@gmail.com

Clinic for Nephrology, University Clinical Center of Sarajevo, Sarajevo, Bosnia and Herzegovina

## References

[1] Vijayan A, Palevsky PM. Dosing of renal replacement therapy in acute kidney injury. Am J Kidney Dis 2012; 59:569–576.

[2] Gabriel DP, Caramori JT, Martin LC, Barretti P, Balbi AL. Continuous peritoneal dialysis compared with daily hemodialysis in patients with acute kidney injury. Perit Dial Int 2009; 29(Suppl. 2):S62–S71.

[3] Gabriel DP, Caramori JT, Martim LC, Barretti P, Balbi AL. High volume peritoneal dialysis vs daily hemodialysis: a randomized, controlled trial in patients with acute kidney injury. Kidney Int Suppl 2008; 108:S87–S93.

[4] Bellomo R, Kellum JA, Ronco C. Acute kidney injury. Lancet 2012; 380:756–766.

[5] Shah BN, Greaves K. The cardiorenal syndrome: a review. Int J Nephrol 2010; 2011:920195.

[6] Cerda J, Bagga A, Kher V, et al. The contrasting characteristics of acute kidney injury in developed and developing countries. Nat Clin Pract Nephrol 2008; 4:138–153.

[7] Kilonzo KG, Ghosh S, Temu SA. Outcome of acute peritoneal dialysis in Northern Tanzania. Perit Dial Int 2012; 32:261–266.

[8] Kumar V, Ramachandran R, Rathi M et al. Peritoneal dialysis: the great savior during disasters. Perit Dial Int 2013; 33:327–329.

[9] Bartal C, Zeller L, Miskin I, et al. Crush syndrome: saving more lives in disasters: lessons learned from the early-response phase in Haiti. Arch Intern Med 2011; 171:694–696.

[10] Cullis B, Abdelraheem M, Abraham G, et al. Peritoneal dialysis for acute kidney injury. ISPD guidelines/recommendations. Perit Dial Int 2014; 34:494–517.

[11] Watcharotone N, Sayumpoorujinant W, Udompon U, et al. Intermittent peritoneal dialysis in acute kidney injury. J Med Assoc Thai 2011; 94:S126–S130.

[12] de Cal M, Cruz DN, Corradi V, et al. HLA-DR expression and apoptosis: a cross-sectional controlled study in hemodialysis and peritoneal dialysis patients. Blood Purif 2008; 26:249–254.

[13] Overberger P, Pesacreta M, Palevsky PM. Management of renal replacement therapy in acute kidney injury: a survey of practitioner prescribing practices. Clin J Am Soc Nephrol 2007; 2:623–630.

[14] Burdmann EA, Chakravarthi R. Peritoneal dialysis in acute kidney injury: lessons learned and applied. Semin Dial 2011; 24:149–156.

[15] Chitalia V, Almeida AF, Rai H, et al. Is peritoneal dialysis adequate for hypercatabolic acute renal failure in developing countries? Kidney Int 2002; 61:747–757.

[16] Ronco C, Kellum JA, Bellomo R, et al. Potential interventions in sepsis-related acute kidney injury. Clin J Am Soc Nephrol 2008; 3:531–544.

[17] Schiffl H. Utility of urea kinetic modelling for prescription of adequate intermittent dialysis in critically ill maintenance dialysis patients. Nephrol Dial Transplant 2007; 22:2096.

[18] Kanagasundaram NS. Prescription of an intermittent haemodialysis dose using urea kinetic modelling is feasible in the critically ill patient. Nephrol Dial Transplant 2008; 23:1075.

[19] Hemodialysis Adequacy 2006 Work Group. Clinical practice guidelines for hemodialysis adequacy, update 2006. Am J Kidney Dis 2006; 48:S2–S90.

[20] Brophy DF, Sowinski KM, Kraus MA, et al. Small and middle molecular weight solute clearance in nocturnal intermittent peritoneal dialysis. Perit Dial Int 1999; 19:534–539.

[21] Bagshaw SM, Brophy PD,Cruz D, et al. Fluid balance as a biomarker: impact of fluid overload on outcome in critically ill patients with acute kidney injury. Crit Care 2008; 12:169.

[22] Krishnan A, Oreopoulos DG. Peritoneal dialysis in congestive heart failure. Adv Perit Dial 2007; 23:82–89.

[23] Mehta RL, Letteri JM. National Kidney Foundation Council on Dialysis: current status on renal replacement therapy for acute renal failure. Am J Nephrol 1999; 19:377–382.

[24] Phu NH, Hien TT, Mai NTH, et al. Hemofiltration and peritoneal dialysis in infection associated acute renal failure in Vietnam. N Engl J Med 2002; 347:895–902.

[25] Gabriel DP, Nascimento GV, Caramori JT, et al. High volume peritoneal dialysis for acute renal failure. Perit Dial Int 2007; 27:277–282.

[26] Roberts M, Ash SR, Lee DBN. Innovative peritoneal dialysis: flow-through and dialysate regeneration. ASAIO J 1999; 45:372–378.

[27] Ponce D, Berbel MN, Regina de Goes C, Almeida CT, Balbi AL. High-volume peritoneal dialysis in acute kidney injury: indications and limitations.Clin J am Soc Nephrol 2012; 7(6):887–894.

[28] Chionh CY, Soni SS, Finkelstein FO, Ronco C, Cruz DN. Use of peritoneal dialysis in AKI: a systematic review. Clin J Am Soc Nephrol. 2013; 8(10):1649–1660.

[29] George J, Varma S, Kumar S, Thomas J, Gopi S, Pisharody R. Comparing continuous venovenous hemodiafiltration and peritoneal dialysis in critically ill patients with acute kidney injury: a pilot study. Perit Dial Int. 2011; 31(4):422–429.

[30] Ponce D, Buffarah MB, Goes C, Balbi A. Peritoneal dialysis in acute kidney injury: trends in the outcome across time periods. PLoS One 2015; 10(5):e0126436. doi: 10.1371/journal.pone.0126436.

[31] Arogundade FA, Ishola DA Jr., Sanusi AA, Akinsola A. An analysis of the effectiveness and benefits of peritoneal dialysis and haemodialysis using Nigerian made PD fluids. Afr J Med Med Sci 2005; 34:227–233.

[32] Thongboonkerd V, Lumlertgul D, Supajatura V. Better correction of metabolic acidosis, blood pressure control, and phagocytosis with bicarbonate compared to lactate solution in acute peritoneal dialysis. Artif Organs 2001; 25:99–108.

[33] Sonnenblick M, Slotki IN, Friedlander Y, Kramer MR. Acute renal failure in the elderly treated by one-time peritoneal dialysis. J Am Geriatr Soc 1988; 36:1039–1044.

[34] Ansari N. Peritoneal dialysis in renal replacement therapy for patients with acute kidney injury. Int J Nephrol 2011; 2011:739794. doi: 10.4061/2011/739794.

[35] Paul TT, Ramprasad KS. Acute peritoneal dialysis using stylet catheter. Saudi J Kidney Dis Transpl. 1994; 5(2):184–189.

[36] Dell'Aquila R, Chiaramonte S, Rodighiero MP, Spanó E, Di Loreto P, Kohn CO, Cruz D, Polanco N, Kuang D, Corradi V, De Cal M, Ronco C. Rational choice of peritoneal dialysis catheter. Perit Dial Int. 2007; 27(Suppl. 2):S119–S125.

[37] Li JR, Chen CH, Chiu KY, Yang CR, Cheng CL, Ou YC, Ko JL, Ho HC. Management of pericannular bleeding after peritoneal dialysis catheter placement. Perit Dial Int. 2012; 32(3):361–362.

[38] Abraham G, Varughese S, Mathew M, Vijayan M. A review of acute and chronic peritoneal dialysis in developing countries. Clin Kidney J. 2015; 8(3):310–317.

[39] Wallace E, Fissell RB, Golper TA, Blake PG, Lewin AM, Oliver MJ, Quinn RR. Catheter insertion and perioperative practices within the ISPD north american research consortium. Perit Dial Int 2015. pii: pdi.2015.00089.

[40] Wong SN, Geary DF. Comparison of temporary and permanent catheters for acute peritoneal dialysis. Arch Dis Child 1988; 63(7):827–831.

[41] Asif A, Tawakol J, Khan T, Vieira CF, Byers P, Gadalean F, Hogan R, Merrill D, Roth D. Modification of the peritoneoscopic technique of peritoneal dialysis catheter insertion: experience of an interventional nephrology program. Semin Dial. 2004; 17(2): 171–173.

[42] Sampathkumar K, Mahaldar AR, Sooraj YS, Ramkrishnan M, Ajeshkumar, Ravichandran R. Percutaneous CAPD catheter insertion by a nephrologist versus surgical placement: a comparative study. Indian J Nephrol 2008; 18(1):5–8.

[43] Al-Hwiesh AK. Percutaneous peritoneal dialysis catheter insertion by a nephrologist: a new simple, and safe technique. Perit Dial Int 2014; 34(2):204–211.

[44] Figueiredo A, Goh BL, Jenkins S, Johnson DW, Mactier R, Ramalakshmi S, Shrestha B, Struijk D, Wilkie M; International Society for Peritoneal Dialysis. Clinical practice guidelines for peritoneal access. Perit Dial Int 2010; 30(4):424–429.

[45] Gadallah MF, Ramdeen G, Mignone J, Patel D, Mitchell L, Tatro S. Role of preoperative antibiotic prophylaxis in preventing postoperative peritonitis in newly placed peritoneal dialysis catheters. Am J Kidney Dis 2000; 36(5):1014–1019.

[46] Strippoli GF, Tong A, Johnson D, Schena FP, Craig JC. Antimicrobial agents for preventing peritonitis in peritoneal dialysis patients. Cochrane Database Syst Rev 2004; 18(4):CD004679.

[47] Nikitidou O, Liakopoulos V, Kiparissi T, Divani M, Leivaditis K, Dombros N. Peritoneal dialysis-related infections recommendations: 2010 update. What is new? Int Urol Nephrol 2012; 44(2):593–600.

[48] Gillerot G, Sempoux C, Pirson Y, Devuyst O. Which type of dialysis in patients with cholesterol crystal embolism? Nephrol Dial Transplant 2002; 17:156–158.

[49] Katz IJ, Sofianou L, Butler O, Hopley M. Recovery of renal function in Black South African patients with malignant hypertension: superiority of continuous ambulatory peritoneal dialysis. Perit Dial Int 2001; 21:581–586.

[50] Chao C-T, Hou C-C, Wu V-C, Lu H-M, Wang C-Y, Chen L, et al. The impact of dialysis-requiring acute kidney injury on long-term prognosis of patients requiring prolonged mechanical ventilation: nationwide population-based study. PLoS One 2012; 7(12):e50675. doi: 10.1371/journal.pone.0050675.

[51] Gupta P, Carlson J, Wells D, Selakovich P, Robertson MJ, Gossett JM, Fontenot EE, Steiner MB. Relationship between renal function and extracorporeal membrane oxygenation use: a single-centre experience. Artif Organs 2015; 39(4):369–374.

[52] Tjiong HL, Rietveld T, Wattimena JL, van den Berg JW, Kahriman D, van der Steen J, Hop WC, Swart R, Fieren MW. Peritoneal dialysis with solutions containing amino acids plus glucose promotes protein synthesis during oral feeding. Clin J Am Soc Nephrol 2007; 2(1):74–80.

[53] Jiang L, Zeng R, Yang K, Mi DH, Tian JH, Ma B, Liu Y. Tidal versus other forms of peritoneal dialysis for acute kidney injury. Cochrane Database Syst Rev 2012; 13(6):CD007016. doi: 10.1002/14651858.CD007016.pub2.

[54] Yong K, Dongra G, Boudville N et al. Acute kidney injury: controversies revisited. Int J Nephrol 2011; 2011:762634.

[55] Sharma RK, Kuma J, Gupta A, Gulati S. Peritoneal infection in acute intermittent peritoneal dialysis. Ren Fail 2003; 25:975–980.

[56] Guest S. Hypoalbuminemia in peritoneal dialysis patients. Adv Perit Dial 2013; 29:55–60.

[57] Chandler WL, Jelacic S, Boster DR, Ciol MA, Williams GD, Watkins SL, Igarashi T, Tarr PI. Prothrombotic coagulation abnormalities preceding the hemolytic-uremic syndrome. N Engl J Med 2002; 346(1):23–32.

[58] Mydlík M, Derzsiová K, Frank K. Renal replacement therapy in acute poisonings—one center experience. Przegl Lek 2013; 70(6):381–385.

[59] Leblanc M, Ouimet D, Pichette V. Dialysate leaks in peritoneal dialysis. Semin Dial 2001; 14(1):50–54.

[60] Piraino B, Sheth H. Peritonitis—does peritoneal dialysis modality make a difference? Blood Purif 2010; 29(2):145–149.

[61] Amerling R, Winchester JF, Ronco C. Continuous flow peritoneal dialysis: update 2012. Contrib Nephrol 2012; 178:205–215.

[62] Bersenas AM. A clinical review of peritoneal dialysis. J Vet Emerg Crit Care (San Antonio) 2011; 21(6):605–617.

[63] Szeto CC. Peritoneal dialysis-related infection in the older population. Perit Dial Int 2015; 35(6):659–662.

[64] Mital S, Fried LF, Piraino B. Bleeding complications associated with peritoneal dialysis catheter insertion. Perit Dial Int 2004; 24(5):478–480.

[65] Dimkovic N. Peritoneal dialysis in acute kidney injury. BANTAO J 2010; 8(2):54–58.

[66] Hayat A, Kamili MA, Samia R, Yaseen M, Shakeel R, Qureshi W, Malik GM. Peritoneal dialysis for adults with acute renal failure: an underutilized modality. Saudi J Kidney Dis Transpl 2007; 18:195–199.

[67] Howdieshell TR, Blalock WE, Bowen PA, Hawkins ML, Hess C. Management of post-traumatic acute renal failure with peritoneal dialysis. Am Surg 1992; 58:378–382.

[68] Ojogwu LI. Peritoneal dialysis in the management of hypertensive acute oliguric renal failure. Trop Geogr Med 1983; 35:385–388.

[69] Cameron JS, Ogg C, Trounce JR. Peritoneal dialysis in hypercatabolic acute renal failure. Lancet 1967; 1:1188–1191.

[70] Chow YW,Lim BB, Hooi LS. Acute renal failure in the same hospital ten years apart. Med J Malaysia 2007; 62:27–32.

[71] Mahajan S, Tiwari S, Bhowmik D, Agarwal SK, Tiwari SC, Dash SC. Factors affecting the outcome of acute renal failure among the elderly population in India: a hospital based study. Int Urol Nephrol 2006; 38:391–396.

[72] Bellomo R, Farmer M, Parkin G, Wright C, Boyce N. Severe acute renal failure: a comparison of acute continuous hemodiafiltration and conventional dialytic therapy. Nephron 1995; 71:59–64.

[73] Hadidy S, Asfari R, Shammaa MZ, Hanifi MI. Acute renal failure among a Syrian population. Incidence, aetiology, treatment and outcome. Int Urol Nephrol 1989; 21:455–461.

[74] Werb R, Linton AL. Aetiology, diagnosis, treatment and prognosis of acute renal failure in an intensive care unit. Resuscitation 1979; 7:95–100.

[75] Ponce D, Dias DB, Nascimento GR, Silveira LV, Balbi AL. Long-term outcome of severe acute kidney injury survivors followed by nephrologists in a developing country. Nephrology (Carlton) 2015. doi: 10.1111/nep.12593. [Epub ahead of print].

[76] Hansson JH, Watnick S. Update on peritoneal dialysis: core curriculum 2016. Am J Kidney Dis 2016; 67(1):151–164.

# Chapter 9

# Peritoneal Dialysis and Pregnancy

Amarpreet S. Sandhu

Additional information is available at the end of the chapter

http://dx.doi.org/10.5772/63474

**Abstract**

Pregnancy is infrequent and has complicated course in women undergoing renal replacement therapy. According to recent data, rates of conception in women on hemodialysis increased from 1.5% to 15% and 1.1% in women on peritoneal dialysis (PD). Lower rates in patients on peritoneal dialysis are due to mechanical factors on top of functional and physiological irregularities. Due to assumption of almost negligible rates of conception, pregnancy symptoms in patients with chronic kidney disease stage V can be confused with uremic symptoms. Once pregnancy is established, multilevel changes need to be made in this patient population. The coordinated care between a nephrologist, obstetrician, and nutritionist is essential for better outcomes. In this chapter, we review a near-missed but a successful case report and details of pregnancy, outcomes, and complications in women on peritoneal dialysis.

**Keywords:** peritoneal dialysis, pregnancy, renal failure, maternal complications, fetal complications

## 1. Introduction

Pregnancy is not only rare but also problematic by maternal and fetal risks and complications in women on dialysis. The first case of female pregnancy while on peritoneal dialysis (PD) was reported in 1980s. The rates of conception in women on peritoneal dialysis are going up but still relatively lower than the rates in women on hemodialysis. Statistically, however, there is no difference in the live birth rate in peritoneal versus hemodialysis women. Due to assumption of almost negligible rates of conception, pregnancy symptoms in patients with chronic kidney disease stage V can be confused with uremic symptoms. In this patient population, basic pregnancy tests are not reliable because most of these markers are cleared by kidneys and can be falsely elevated. For better outcomes, a multilevel coordinated care is needed for pregnant women on renal replacement therapy.

## 2. Prevalence

Although conception in end-stage renal disease (ESRD) patients is infrequent, recent data show that the conception rates are improving overtime. According to data from Registry of Pregnancy in Dialysis Patients (RPDP), conception rate in hemodialysis patients over a 4-year period (1992–1995) is 2.4%, whereas it was 1.5% in a 2-year period (1990–1992) in the past [1, 2]. Although most pregnancies in this patient population occur during the first few years on dialysis, there are case reports of pregnancies in women who were on dialysis for as long as 20 years. Repeated pregnancies are also not unknown. Out of 353 pregnant women reported by RPDP, eight became pregnant three times, eight became pregnant twice, and one became pregnant four times [1].

Saudi Arabia dialysis unit questionnaire data reported improved pregnancy rates of 5–7.9% [3, 4]. The Canada reported data with conception rate of 15.9% in women on intensive nocturnal hemodialysis [5]. Pregnancy in peritoneal dialysis patients remains low. According to data collection from 1699, in childbearing-age women on peritoneal dialysis, conception rate is only 1.1% [1].

## 3. Conception

Menstrual irregularities, infertility, and sexual dysfunction are known to occur in end-stage renal disease (ESRD) patients, and these functional and physiological abnormalities worsen as renal disease progresses. Holley et al. [6] described this parallel relationship where menstrual cycle irregularities begin when estimated glomerular filtration rate (eGFR) fall below 15 ml/min/1.73 $m^2$ and progresses to amenorrhea at eGFR below 5 ml/min/1.73 $m^2$.

Hormonal abnormality studies in dialysis patients observed an anovulatroy cycles even in menstruating women. In 70–90% of the women, progesterone and estradiol hormone levels are low, whereas prolactin levels are high. Luteinizing hormone (LH) levels are elevated and follicular-stimulating hormone (FSH) levels are same or slightly lower to levels in normal women during the follicular phase of menstrual cycle. Although LH levels in women on dialysis are elevated, they fail to have luteal surge of LH, which is directly related to ovulation [7, 8]. Many other fertility-affecting factors in ESRD patients include subclinical hypothyroidism, medications, fatigue, anemia, and depression, which further results in lack of libido [9–11].

Furthermore, lower conception rate in patients on peritoneal dialysis are also due to mechanical factor. Recurrent peritonitis can also lead to fallopian tube obstruction. It is possible that hypertonic dextrose (dextrose dialysate solution) damages the ovum, or the volume to dialysate in the peritoneal space interferes with ovum transfer within the fallopian tube [12].

http://dx.doi.org/10.5772/63474

## 4. Diagnosis

Menstrual irregularities and amenorrhea challenge and delay the diagnosis of pregnancy in ESRD women. Human chorionic gonadotropin (HCG) is partially cleared by the kidneys and results in false-positive serum pregnancy tests in ESRD women. Beta-hCG and maternal serum pregnancy-associated plasma protein A (PAPP-A) are generally elevated in ESRD patients because these are inversely correlated with creatinine clearance. Hence, careful interpretation of these tests is advised while screening these women in the first trimester [11, 13, 14].

Therefore, among women suspected of pregnancy should be evaluated by ultrasonography to verify presence of viable fetus and to obtain the approximate gestational age. All confirmed pregnant women should be referred to high-risk obstetrician.

## 5. Case discussion

There have been multiple case reports of pregnancy in women on peritoneal and hemodialysis. Here, I present my published case to illustrate pregnancy diagnosis difficulty and management in women on peritoneal dialysis.

A 25 years old female with past medical history of hypertension, optic neuritis, history of pyelonephritis, left middle cranial fossa arachnoid cyst, asthma, and end-stage renal disease (ESRD) secondary to autosomal dominant polycystic kidney disease (ADPKD) was transferred to renal clinic with concerning uremic symptoms with nausea, anorexia, and loss of weight. Her medications included diovan, oxycodone, Phenergan, calcium with vitamin D. At the time of presentation to renal clinic, her serum creatinine was 2.7 and estimated glomerular filtration rate (eGFR) of 26 ml/min/1.73 m$^2$. Given low chances of conception in ESRD patients, false-positive beta human chorionic gonadotropin (β-HCG) test in this patient population, no concern of pregnancy by patient, and previously unremarkable ultrasound other than ADPKD her symptoms were thought to be due to uremia. After discussion, the patient elected to have a peritoneal dialysis. A PD catheter was placed and she was referred to PD clinic for education, training, and initiation of PD.

Two weeks later, she presented to the emergency room with persistent symptoms of nausea, vomiting, and now abdominal cramps. A computerized tomography (CT) scan of abdomen and pelvis revealed ascending colitis probably inflammatory versus infectious, scattered free intra-abdominal fluid, but no documentation of uterus. Given low concerns of pregnancy, β-HCG test was not obtained and she was discharged with the diagnosis of the gastroenteritis. Even after a month of initiation of PD, patient continued to have nausea, vomiting, and anorexia and her dialysis exchanges were increased to 5/day and calcium supplements were discontinued. Her first dialysis adequacy (Kt/V) was 3.2.

Given persistent symptoms of nausea and vomiting, she was referred to her primary care physician (PCP) for further workup. A pregnancy test with β-HCG was positive, which could be falsely positive because β-HCG is partially cleared by kidneys. Due to high suspicious for pregnancy, her diovan was immediately stopped and started on labetalol for hypertension management. Obstetrics ultrasound revealed 20 weeks of pregnancy and she was referred to the obstetrician for close follow-up. Thereafter, she continued to have coordinated care by her nephrologist, obstetrician, and nutritionist.

Her dialysis adequacy was maintained with Kt/V urea of >3.0 and blood urea nitrogen (BUN) <50 throughout the pregnancy (**Figures 1** and **2**). She was treated with increased doses of Epogen and iron for anemia and calcitriol for secondary hyperparathyroidism. Her pregnancy remained uneventful and she continued her PD until 38 weeks and 5 days of gestation when she presented to the hospital because she was unable to perform her peritoneal dialysis (PD) for 4 days due to abdominal discomfort.

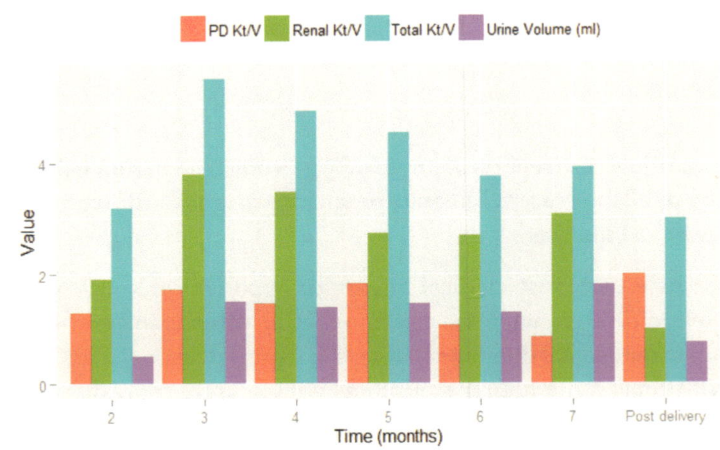


**Figure 1.** Kt/V and urine volume measurement in a woman on peritoneal dialysis during pregnancy.

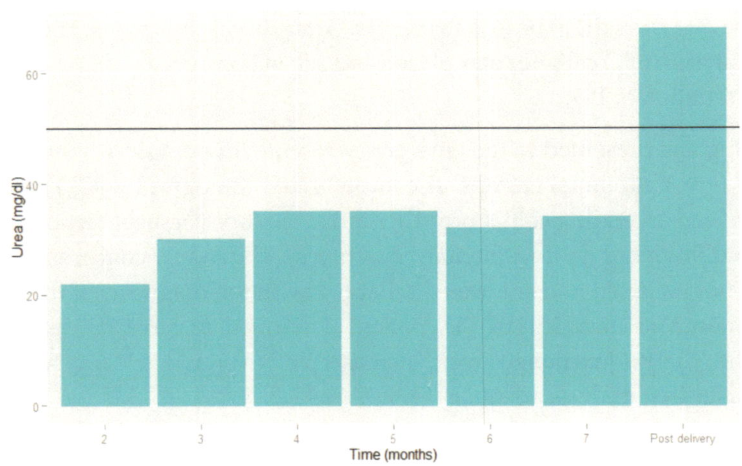


**Figure 2.** BUN measurement in a woman on peritoneal dialysis during pregnancy.

Since patient was not able to continue PD, an option of hemodialysis was discussed with the patient. She declined to start on the hemodialysis, rather chose an induction of labor for delivery. PD was continued with small frequent exchanges during labor. A healthy baby was delivered with uneventful postpartum period. Regular PD prescription was resumed 12 h after delivery. She was discharged to home 3 days after delivery [11].

## 6. Drug therapy

The physicians need to be very careful of medications used to treat kidney disease in pregnant women. It is also important to evaluate medication risk on fetus. Since most common antihypertensive medicines such as angiotensin-converting enzyme inhibitors and angiotensin II receptor blockers are associated with neonatal morbidity and mortality, these should be discontinued. Alternative antihypertensives such as β-blockers and hydralazine are relatively safe during pregnancy.

## 7. General obstetrical management

As mentioned earlier, all women with diagnosis of pregnancy while on dialysis should be referred to high-risk obstetrician. Some of the general guidelines that high-risk obstetrician follows include increased frequency of prenatal visits, early detection and treatment of asymptomatic bacteriuria, detect early signs of preeclampsia, frequent fetal surveillance, and preterm intervention or induction of labor.

## 8. General nephrology management

All nephrologists needs to be aware that although low risk but women on dialysis can become pregnant. The differentiation of uremic and pregnancy symptoms is the key. Early detected pregnant dialysis women should receive a multilevel coordinated care.

Some of the general guidelines include increased frequency of dialysis, BUN goal <50 mg/dl, target Kt/V goal of 2.2–2.4, increased doses of potassium supplements, Epogen, and iron, and maintain adequate volume and weight.

## 9. Maternal risks and complications

The maternal complications include premature birth, uncontrolled hypertension, miscarriage, placental detachment, anemia, and infection, premature rupture of membranes, polyhydramnios, preeclampsia, eclampsia, hemorrhage, C-section, and even maternal death.

### 9.1. Premature birth

According to RPDP reported birth in women on dialysis, 84% of infants were born prematurely, 44% weighed less than 1500 g, and 28% were small for gestational age. Gestational age of survived infants f women on peritoneal dialysis ranged from 31 to 38 weeks [1].

### 9.2. Hypertension

Hypertension in pregnant dialysis patients is very common. Approximately, 80% of pregnant dialysis women have a blood pressure (BP) higher than 140/90 and even more than 50% have BP greater than 170/110. Given continuous therapy in PD to achieve euvolemic status, it is thought that PD patient should have lower risk of hypertension, but small studies have shown no difference [11, 12]. Since hypertension in dialysis patients is mostly related to their volume status, it poses another challenge to determine dry weight in pregnant dialysis women (see below for details).

### 9.3. Preeclampsia/eclampsia/HELLP syndrome

Preeclampsia is when pregnant women develop high blood pressure and a significant amount of protein in the urine after the 20th week (i.e., late second or third trimester) of pregnancy. If left untreated, it can lead to an acute and life-threatening condition with tonic-clonic seizures, called eclampsia. HELLP syndrome is identified with a group of hematological alterations including hemolysis, elevated liver enzymes, and low platelet count. In 10–20% of the cases, HELLP can occur as a complication in women with severe preeclampsia or eclampsia [15].

Preeclampsia is difficult to diagnose in dialysis patients due to anuria that makes unable to determine proteinuria. In these patients, preeclampsia diagnosis relies on the assessment of worsening blood pressure, fetal growth retardation, alterations in placental Doppler blood flow and hematological abnormalities in case of HELLP syndrome [11, 15].

### 9.4. Urea clearance, dialysis adequacy, and polyhydramnios

In pregnant women on dialysis, blood urea nitrogen (BUN) level is an important marker of overall fetal outcome. Many isolated clinical cases and retrospective studies have reported improved fetal survival in women with BUN <50 mg/dl. Increased frequency of dialysis to four to six sessions per week to achieve at least 20 h of dialysis per week helps to keep BUN goal <50 mg/dl [16, 17]. It also helps better control of hypertension, improves maternal nutrition, and prevents polyhydramnios [11].

There is no commonly accepted target Kt/V for pregnant PD patients. However, Okundaye and Hou [18] has reported target Kt/V goal of 2.2–2.4 for better outcomes. Higher Kt/V is achieved by increasing fill volume that might be difficult in pregnant patients due to discomfort. Intensive PD is very important in the third trimester when fetal urea production is increased to 540 mg/day. This can be achieved by increasing small volume exchanges as we did in our reported patient.

Approximately, 30–70% pregnant dialysis women have incidence of polyhydramnios. Due to urea-induced osmotic diuresis there is increased production in fetal urine that further leads to excess amniotic fluid. Increased dialysis dose in this patient population can help reduce these complications [19, 20].

### 9.5. Electrolytes, vitamins, minerals, and acid-base abnormalities

Most of the electrolytes abnormalities occur due to increased dialysis dose in these patients. Hypokalemia gets worse in dialyzed pregnant PD patient that requires increased doses of potassium supplementation. Usually, phosphate binders are discontinued in hemodialysis patients. Phosphate replacement might be needed in pregnant PD patients [11, 18].

Minerals and water soluble vitamins are often removed by intensive dialysis and usually require double the dose of daily multivitamins, particularly folic acid. The pregnant PD women do not have metabolic alkalosis that is usually seen in hemodialysis patients and requires lower bicarbonate bath to maintain normal physiological bicarbonate goal of 25 meq/L [12].

### 9.6. Anemia

The etiology of anemia in pregnant dialysis women is multifactorial including erythropoietin resistance probably from pregnancy induced cytokines, high demand of red blood cell production for fetal growth, and the iron and red blood cell loss from intense frequent dialysis. Therefore, iron requirement increases to 30 mg/day and erythropoietin requirement increases by 50% [5].

### 9.7. Nutrition and weight gain

Nutritional assessment and counseling is very important to ensure adequate protein and caloric intake. Adequate protein intake might be difficult in this patient population due to nausea, anorexia, and protein loss due to intensive dialysis. The pregnant dialysis women should take in 1 g/kg/day protein, adding 20 g/day for fetal growth [21]. For development of fetal skeleton, maternal diet should include an additional 30 g of calcium supplementation [12].

Weight gain determination in pregnant dialysis patient is very difficult. About 9 L of total body water increases in pregnancy that leads to intravascular expansion due to vasodilatation, making fluid removal difficult. The pregnant mother should gain a minimum of 1–1.5 kg in the first trimester and 0.45–1 kg/week afterward [17]. Estimated dry weight (EDW) should be increased to 400 g/week after first trimester to account for fetal weight of about 500 mg/week in the second and third trimester [20]. A pregnant woman with a normal body mass index should gain maternal weight of 11–15 kg [11].

### 9.8. Peritonitis and bloody effluent

There is limited information on peritonitis in pregnant CAPD patients. In three reported cases of peritonitis in pregnant PD patients, labor occurred in two women. One resulted in still birth and other in premature baby who survived [18]. RPDP reported that five out of six pregnancies which were complicated by peritonitis, resulted in surviving infants. One woman had second trimester spontaneous abortion. There is always risk of peritonitis from any pregnancy-associated infections due to connection between peritoneum and fallopian tubes. Cephalosporins and penicillins are safe antibiotics to use in pregnancy associated peritonitis [18].

In nonpregnant PD patients, bloody effluent is rarely a sign of a serious problem. However, it is concerning in pregnant PD patients and can indicate impending abortion or placental abruption [22]. These patients should be hospitalized for observation and placental separation should be ruled out with fetal ultrasound [11].

### 9.9. Anticoagulation

Heparin does not cross the placenta and is not teratogenic. Low molecular weight heparin (LMWH) appears to be as safe as unfractionated heparin (UH) in pregnant women. LMWH has a favorable dosing route and interval and requires less monitoring than UH. Therefore, it can be safely used in pregnant women to prevent access clotting in HD and to maintain fibrin free dialysis in PD. Coumadin is contraindicated in these patients [11, 23].

### 9.10. Labor and delivery

At the time of labor and delivery especially in cases of preeclampsia magnesium is given in high doses. In this patient population, magnesium must be administered with caution and maintain magnesium levels below 5–7 mg/dl to prevent toxicity [23].

Dialysis status by itself does not warrant for C-section. However, if required for obstetric reasons, C-section can be performed successfully in PD patients. The abdomen should be drained before surgery and if it is possible surgery should be done extraperitoneally. In 24 h after the surgery, peritoneal dialysis can be resumed with small volume exchanges. In cases of PD fluid leakage, patients should be switched to hemodialysis for 2 weeks [11, 12].

## 10. Fetal risks and complications

All infants born to women on dialysis should be observed in high-risk setting. Major complications in the newborn are due to growth retardation and prematurity.

Neonates born with BUN and serum Cr same as of their mother's serum BUN and Cr which leads to osmotic diuresis and can cause significant volume contraction and electrolytes imbalance if losses are not replaced. Several retrospective studies and clinical cases have reported increased fetal survival in women with BUN <50 mg/dl. Breast milk will have high concentration of urea and in cases of breast-feeding it can lead to osmotic diuresis in these infants [11, 18].

Infants who are exposed to hypercalcemia during pregnancy are at increased risk of hypocalcemia and tetany after birth [12].

## 11. Overall outcomes

In a series, Redrow et al. [22] concluded that peritoneal dialysis is superior to hemodialysis. However, data reported by them did not support this conclusion. According to an early report by RPDP, there is no statistical difference in the live birth rate in peritoneal (47.6%) versus hemodialysis (46.4%) patients [1]. In a single center study, Chow et al. reported worse outcomes in peritoneal dialysis patients [24]. Theoretically, peritoneal dialysis is considered superior to hemodialysis for pregnancy given more stable biochemical parameters, higher mean hemoglobin, gentle daily ultrafiltration, and no required systemic anticoagulation [25].

## 12. Conclusion

The rates of pregnancy in ESRD women are increasing overtime. Besides the challenges of functional and physiological irregularities seen in hemodialysis patients, PD women also face mechanical challenges. Most of the patients who get pregnant while on PD are transitioned to daily HD during pregnancy with the goals of keeping their BUN <50 mg/dl and spKt/V > 2.2–2.4. However, the live birth rate not different between PD (47.6%) and HD (46.4%) receiving women. A highly coordinate care between patient, her nephrologist obstetrician, neonatologist, dialysis nurse, and her nutritionist is essential for better outcome.

## Author details

Amarpreet S. Sandhu

Address all correspondence to: Sandhudoctor@gmail.com

Department of Transplantation, California Pacific Medical Center, San Francisco, California, USA

## References

[1] Okundaye I, Abrinko P, Hou S. Registry of pregnancy in dialysis patients. Am J Kidney Dis 1998;31:766–773.

[2] Hou SH. Frequency and outcome of pregnancy in women on dialysis. Am J Kidney Dis 1994;23:60–63.

[3] Malik GH, Al-Harbi A, Al-Mohaya S, Dohaimi H, Kechrid M, Shetaia MS, Al-Hassan AO, Quiapos LS. Pregnancy in patients on dialysis—experience at a referral center. J Assoc Physicians India 2005;53:937–941.

[4] Bahloul H, Kammoun K, Kharrat M, Jarraya F, Charffedine K, Hamida MB, Hachicha J. Pregnancy in chronic hemodialysis women: outcome of multicentric study. Saudi J Kidney Dis Transpl 2003;14:530–531.

[5] Barua M, Hladunewich M, Keunen J, Pierratos A, McFarlane P, Sood M, Chan CT. Successful pregnancies on nocturnal home hemodialysis. Clin J Am Soc Nephrol 2008;3:392–396.

[6] Holley JL, Schmidt RJ, Bender FH, Dumler F, Schiff M. Gynecologic and reproductive issues in women on dialysis. Am J Kidney Dis 1997;29:685–690.

[7] Lim VS, Henriquez C, Sievertsen G, Frohman LA. Ovarian function in chronic renal failure. Evidence of hypothalamic anovulation. Ann Intern Med 1980;93:21–27.

[8] Lim VS, Kathpalia SC, Frohman LA. Hyperprolactinemia and impaired pituitary response to suppression and stimulation in chronic renal failure: reversal after transplantation. J Clin Endocrinol Metab 1979;48:101–107.

[9] Bailie GR, Elder SJ, Mason NA, Asano Y, Cruz JM, Fukuhara S, Lopes AA, Mapes DL, Mendelssohn DC, Bommer J, Young EW. Sexual dysfunction in dialysis patients treated with antihypertensive or antidepressive medications: results from the DOPPS. Nephrol Dial Transplant 2007;22:1163–1170.

[10] Steele TE, Wuerth D, Finkelstein S, Juergensen D, Juergensen P, Kliger AS, Finkelstein FO. Sexual experience of the chronic peritoneal dialysis patient. J Am Soc Nephrol 1996;7:1165–1168.

[11] Sandhu A, Regmi A, Buchwald D, et al. Pregnancy or Uremia? – case report and review of conception, pregnancy, and complications in peritoneal dialysis patients. Cureus 2014;6(9):e206.

[12] Hou S. Conception and pregnancy in peritoneal dialysis patients. Perit Dial Int 2001;21:S290–S294.

[13] Buckner CL, Wilson L, Papadea CN. An unusual cause of elevated serum total beta hCG. Ann Clin Lab Sci 2007;37:186–191.

[14] Shenhav S, Gemer O, Sherman DJ, Peled R, Segal S. Midtrimester triple-test levels in women with chronic hypertension and altered renal function. Prenat Diagn 2003;23:166–167.

[15] Hladunewich M, Hercz AE, Keunen J, Chan C, Pierratos A. Pregnancy in end stage renal disease. Semin Dial 2011;24(6):634–639.

[16] Asamiya Y, Otsubo S, Matsuda Y, Kimata N, Kikuchi K, Miwa N, et al. The importance of low blood urea nitrogen levels in pregnant patients undergoing hemodialysis to optimize birth weight and gestational age. Kidney Int 2009;75(11):1217–1222.

[17] Giatras I, Levy DP, Malone FD, Carlson JA, Jungers P. Pregnancy during dialysis: case report and management guidelines. Nephrol Dial Transplant 1998;13:3266–3272.

[18] Okundaye I, Hou S. Management of pregnancy in women undergoing continuous ambulatory peritoneal dialysis. Adv Perit Dial 1996;12:151–155.

[19] Haase M, Morgera S, Bamberg CH, Halle H, Martini S, Hocher B, et al. A systematic approach to managing pregnant dialysis patients—the importance of an intensified haemodiafiltration protocol. Nephrol Dial Transplant 2005;20:2537–2542.

[20] Luders C, Castro MC, Titan SM, De Castro I, Elias RM, Abensur H, et al. Obstetric outcome in pregnant women on long-term dialysis: a case series. Am J Kidney Dis 2010;56(1):77–85.

[21] Ikizler TA, Flakoll PJ, Parker RA, Hakim RM. Amino acid and albumin losses during hemodialysis. Kidney Int 1994;46:830–837.

[22] Redrow M, Cherem L, Elliot J, Mangalat J, Mishler RE, Bennet WM, et al. Dialysis in the management of pregnant patients with renal insufficiency. Medicine 1988;67:199–208.

[23] Vázquez-Rodríguez JG. Hemodialysis and pregnancy: technical aspects. Cir Cir 2010;78(1):99–102.

[24] Chou CY, Ting IW, Lin TH, Lee CN. Pregnancy in patients on chronic dialysis: a single center experience and combined analysis of reported results. Eur J Obstet Gynecol Reprod Biol 2008;136:165–170.

[25] Lew SQ, Watson JA. Urea and creatinine generation and removal in a pregnant patient receiving peritoneal dialysis. Adv Perit Dial 1992;8:131–135.